Dear Ca...

Sara,
Beyond the Veil

I hope this book
brings you Peace.

Rev. Susan Hurley

Sara, Beyond the Veil

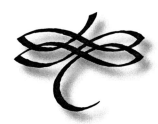

A Spiritual Look at Dementia

REV. SUSAN J. HENLEY

BALBOA
PRESS

A DIVISION OF HAY HOUSE

ISBN: 978-1-4525-6085-4 (sc)
ISBN: 978-1-4525-6087-8 (hc)
ISBN: 978-1-4525-6086-1 (e)

Library of Congress Control Number: 2012920047

Balboa Press books may be ordered through booksellers or by contacting:

Balboa Press
A Division of Hay House
1663 Liberty Drive
Bloomington, IN 47403
www.balboapress.com
1-(877) 407-4847

Printed in the United States of America

Balboa Press rev. date: 10/18/2012

Preface

The inspiration for this story came from my Aunt Sara. She was one of the kindest women I know. Before she passed away she began to drift from us. She had fallen and was confined to a wheel chair. Sara was living in a residential nursing home and the last thing she said to me was "I wish you'd take me out of here." I would visit a few times a week, sitting for hours with her watching television. She would just stare, not say anything and seem to be in her own world; a world no one could enter. It was because of her, this story began to unfold. The Sara in this book is not my Aunt Sara, but I hope that the sweetness of who she was comes through in some of the pages.

My late husband, Larry, provided me with the character of Peter. My hope is that I have honored him in a way that he would be proud. He was amazing, showing great courage in the face of suffering. He came back to God while in the midst of a battle with cancer that he eventually lost, but his Soul was not. He found the meadow.

While I was never sure of Sara's diagnosis, I have seen many people who suffer from dementia. It places a great burden on the people who are suffering and their caregivers. Pressures can be social, economical and psychological. Parenting your parent becomes necessary as the roles we partake in become reversed.

My firm belief is that just because someone has died, the relationship never ends. If someone you love goes on a trip, because they are across the country, or even on another continent, the relationship continues. People who have lost loved ones will smell their perfume or aftershave, feel as though someone is touching their shoulder or caressing their hair. This indicates the relationship continues. Sometimes being in an altered state allows us to be more aware of that which is unseen.

This book is about life and death, and incorporates experiences that I have had with those who honored me by allowing me to be with them when they died. To be there, at the moment when life moves from the physical body to the Body of the Divine, is an amazing experience. One day it will be my turn, but until then it is my hope that I can be of service to those who don't know about The Veil, or beyond it.

Acknowledgements

First I need to thank my son Sean for catapulting me forward in my Spiritual growth. If not for his passing, I would still be reading and not doing. I want to thank my daughter, Somer Healey for her amazing creativity in designing the cover of this book and her sweet editing. To Becky Harris for believing in me and moving me forward. To Pastor Peter Perry for giving me an incredible look at how God sees time and his kind words about dementia patients. To my Mom, Georgiana Blume, for listening to me ramble for years about getting this book out. To my Spiritual Teachers who provided me with knowledge and experiences that enabled me to see Beyond the Veil. To my friends, family and colleagues that sat patiently while I went on and on about how this book would be done "very soon" and smiled, knowing that someday I really would finish it!

Chapter 1

When Peter and Sara met, he was overwhelmed with feelings he had never had before. His heart started racing and sweat formed on his brow. With his knees buckling slightly, he felt a chill run through his entire body. He could not believe what he saw in her eyes. When he first looked into them he lost himself. He couldn't speak or barely breathe for what seemed like minutes. Where had this beautiful woman been and why hadn't he seen her before; or had he?

Sara immediately knew who Peter was. She had dreamed of him again and again throughout her life and he was exactly as she had seen him. His voice sounded as it had, he was dressed in the same flannel shirt and jeans, his deep blue eyes and sandy blond hair showed his Norwegian descent. He was tall with square shoulders to match his square jaw.

It was a beautiful day, the fall breeze had begun and people felt they could step outside and enjoy the day. It had been a long and grueling summer in the city and the Farmers Market in downtown Phoenix welcomed visitors and natives alike. Small groups of people were milling around, talking quietly, and sampling the fresh popped popcorn and roasted almonds.

Her dog Buster saw Peter too. They were standing at a local fruit stand eying the red delicious apples. Buster, a medium black and white mix, started to wag his tail and whine. He pulled on his leash as Peter knelt down a few feet away to welcome him. Sara couldn't help but follow.

"Hey, boy, isn't this an amazing day?" he said. His voice was powerful but gentle.

That's the voice from my dreams, she thought.

Peter gazed up at Sara. *Where has this beautiful woman been and why haven't I seen her before, or have I?*

There was something so familiar about Sara. Maybe it was the scent of her perfume or the time on the beach where he attended a wedding in Hawaii. Or maybe was it the time when he was hiking in Sedona? This resonated with him in a place deep inside; a place he could not explain and had not felt in this lifetime.

Sara was short in stature with eyes so dark brown you could barely see the iris. Her hair matched her eyes, and she typically wore it up with little strands falling around her shoulders. Her dress was contemporary and always showed her beautiful Italian figure.

Everything about this man standing in front of her was the man she had dreamed of. She just hadn't known his name. Now here he was, stepping all over his words as he was trying to say what had been said in her dreams.

"Hu, hullo…how, how, ah, my na…., oh my," was all he could get out.

Sara smiled, and as she did her eyes glistened with recognition and love. Finally, he was here. Why had it taken so long?

"I've been waiting for you," she said.

He looked at her somewhat puzzled. "Waiting?"

"I mean I've seen you before," she quickly corrected herself.

"Oh? Where?" he asked, trying to get his thoughts together while she talked. Surely he would remember seeing someone this beautiful before. It wouldn't make sense that he didn't remember her.

"On the docks in Monterrey, I think," she tried to think of something fast. "My name is Sara Russo. What's yours?" She reached out to him with her right hand, trying to distract him from her earlier misstep.

"Peter Hansen," timidly he stretched his hand out to shake hers as he stood to face her.

She touched his hand with such softness and he almost melted. There was a strange yet familiar feeling enveloping him as soon as he felt her. It was warm and comforting, loving and tender. He almost asked her to marry him right then.

Sara's beauty and grace moved him like no other. His first instinct was to back away, not get involved; but the glow of her presence and the touch of her hand made him move forward, expecting the unexpected happiness which had eluded him his entire life.

"I deserve her," he thought.

While he was a good man, always kind to those around him, he never grasped the concept of good things being available to him. Peter rarely thought he deserved much at all. He acknowledged a gentle nudge on his shoulder moving him towards her and decided this must be right. He glanced behind him but didn't see anyone there.

After their first touch they were as comfortable as if they had been together for years. They walked in silence holding hands. Neither knew where they were going; only they would now be together. It was exactly the way it was supposed to be, the continuation of their journey, picking up from where it had left off lifetimes ago. The familiarity, the knowingness, the love.

He felt Buster nudge against his leg and he moved closer to Sara.

This must be right.

Sara smiled. Her eyes glistened with recognition and love.

Finally, he's here. What's taken so long? I'm not going to ask anymore. I just glad he's here.

Their courtship was quick and soon they decided to marry. Both of their parents protested, saying they hardly knew each other. Sara's mother was the most vocal.

"How can you marry this boy? You don't know him; you only met him a month ago. What if he turns out to be some kind of ax murderer?" Sara's mother Rosa exclaimed. "Do you even know what kind of family he comes from? And he's a smoker! How can you be with someone who smokes? I'll bet he's an atheist."

Rosa's family had come from Italy and they believed she should marry only an Italian/Catholic man. She'd had a hard life, working as a cleaning lady for a very rich family. She was short like Sara, but with a few extra pounds. Her gray hair was pulled tight in a bun and she was always wearing an apron.

"Mother! For goodness sakes. I've been dreaming about him for years. He's the one I told you about. You never believed me and yet here he is. I'm going to marry him whether you like it or not!" Sara stomped out of the room and out the front door. She sat on the steps with her arms crossed and her head on her knees.

"You're only 21 you know." It was her dad. Paul Russo had worked on the docks in Italy and California all his life, and it showed. His hair was grey, cut neatly to his neck. Broad shoulders filled his flannel long-sleeve shirt, covering his muscular arms. Paul moved his family to Phoenix when Sara became sick with allergies. Here he was able to find work at a local grocery store's warehouse, driving a fork lift and he always did his job well. Devoted to his job; devoted to his family.

"I know how old I am Dad; you don't have to remind me." Sara voice was filled with sarcasm. "It's just that he's The One!"

"Why don't we meet his parents? Have Momma cook a nice dinner, huh? We'll have them over and get to know everyone. That will make Momma feel better." Paul was always trying to keep the peace, and he had become quite good at it over the years.

"Alright, I'll ask him, but everyone has to be on their best behavior. No asking questions about religion or how much money they make," Sara demanded.

Sara set the ground rules and everyone, even Rosa for a change, followed them. The dinner went well and the parents on both sides decided with some reservations, the marriage was right. It was time for Sara and Peter to get married and start their life together.

The wedding was at St. Frances, a beautiful Catholic church in north Phoenix. Peter had been raised Lutheran though he no longer attended services. Neither Peter nor Sara really cared where they married; just being able to say their vows and move forward with their life together was the goal. It was a traditional ceremony for the sake of Sara's parents; however, Peter and Sara wrote their own vows. When it came time to read them they faced each other and spoke, taking turns. Everyone was moved.

"My promise to you is but a simple one," Peter smiled as he looked into her eyes.

"I will love you today and every day after until the end of time," Sara smiled in return.

"With the passing of every minute, my love and devotion grows stronger and grows deeper."

"I will love and cherish you until my ears can no longer hear." She took his hands in hers.

"I will love and cherish you until my eyes can no longer see." He gently squeezed her hands.

"I will love and cherish you until my hands can no longer feel."

"From this moment until my dying breath, you are my love. You are my life."

"From this moment until my dying breath, you are my love. You are my life." Sara embraced him with the last line of their vows.

They spent their honeymoon in Sedona, Arizona, a beautiful, breathtaking community which offered hiking, horseback riding and more. This was considered a New Age community. The melding of red, yellow and orange sandstone filled the area and the spectacular images made their honeymoon much more special. Buster was welcome at the hotel where they stayed and he went on hikes with them in the mountains and by the creek. Everywhere they went; they held hands or had their arms around each other. The soft, sweet touch of her hand in his gave him strength and a peace he had never felt before. This place gave Peter the sense of belonging, a sense of connection to the earth and to a higher source. Sara too was touched by the area, but her strong religious background limited her from opening up to the expansive energy of the place.

She was curious about spirits and the after-life. This place provided a variety of different options to research and observe. For Sara, it had too many different beliefs, which made it difficult for her to choose one. Peter just "went with the flow" of whoever he was talking with or whatever he ran across.

After they were married for a few years, Sara became interested in the Lutheran way, feeling it may be a little more lenient, less restrictive than what she was used to. She joined St. Johns, a local Lutheran church where she felt at home. Peter didn't attend as frequently as Sara, but he would go on holidays. She found contentment and friendship in this lovely church. Little did she know her beliefs would be challenged over time.

Chapter 2

At 32, Brian, Sara and Peter's older child, was tall like his father with his father's eyes and his mother's hair. He was strikingly handsome and very successful in his marketing career. So successful he didn't allow himself to have time for a wife and family of his own. Life had become about possessions, he had already obtained everything a man could want. He just couldn't commit to a long-term relationship, after having been hurt by who he considered to be "the one." Brian wanted to marry this woman, and they even had a child together, but she cheated on him with his best friend and it was too much for him. Because of this, he became conflicted about starting a family. So for him it was just easier to retreat into his work and have short or distant relationships. A relationship which required little commitment wouldn't hurt so much.

Brian had no beliefs in an afterlife. Sara had talked about spirits all his life, but he needed to have experiences for him to belief. He was a "seeing is believing" type of guy, and he just hadn't seen. It was easier for him to think of spirituality as a lot of hype to make people feel good about what wasn't there. Science had not proven anything about life after death, and this made him uneasy about having any discussions not proven to his satisfaction.

Emma, Sara and Peter's daughter, on the other hand, was a believer. Emma was taller than her mother, with dark eyes and dark hair and loved to dress in bright peach and light blue colors. She was of slim build and had a walk of confidence. Three years younger than Brian, she could hold her own with anyone; assertive but not aggressive. She read every book she could find on spirits, the paranormal and metaphysics. She was fixated on life after death. Every time someone came to the local library to speak on the subject, Emma was there. If a movie came out about the paranormal she was first in line to see it.

Emma had married Tom Huston, who was career military. He joined the Army straight out of high school. Tom traveled from base to base and Emma always went with him until she gave birth to their little girl Emily. They were in their late twenties by this time, having traveled to a few different countries, living on base and sometimes off, depending on what country they were in. Emily had been ill when she was a few months old and spent many months in and out of the base hospital.

Sara and Peter travelled to Clarksville, Tennessee a few days before Emily arrived to be there when she was born. "You know she said Papa when I first saw her in the hospital," Peter would tease. "That was her first word. She wasn't even an hour old when I held her. She clearly said Papa!"

Emily was born nearly a month early, and not quite fully developed. After the first few weeks of non-stop visits to the hospital and frustration, Emma decided to move back to Phoenix to be closer to her parents. She needed the support only her mother could give. They could help her while Tom had to be overseas for months at a time. While Tom was saddened by the thought of them moving away, he supported her decision, knowing it would be the best for all of them in the long run.

The Children's Hospital in Phoenix was the best in the country. There Emily received quality care and Emma received the comfort and support of the great staff, along with the support of her parents. Emily began to grow fast after the age of two and soon talked all the time. She had her own language Peter understood.

"Banna, banna. Oook, Papa, ook. Dare dare dare!" Emily was pointing to the big picture window facing the back yard as if she saw something there.

"What, Em? I don't see anything," Peter looked playfully out of the window.

He was Papa to her and she was Em to him. They had become very close over the last few years. Peter would go to the hospital and sit with Emily in his lap for hours as she slept. Her light blond hair was growing long and straight. Her blue eyes were so beautiful and very hard for anyone to resist. The nurses adored her. Even though she may have appeared to have a slow start, she was catching up fast.

"Papa, dey rite dare!" she screamed. "Dey rite dare!"

By now she was nearly five and running everywhere. She jumped off of Peter's lap, ran to the window and began having a conversation with someone Peter couldn't see. This went on for 15 minutes before she moved on to her toys.

Em would speak as though she were asking a question and then pause, appear to get an answer and start speaking again. Even though Peter couldn't see anything or anyone, this wasn't the first time Emily had done this. It was becoming a ritual for her to have conversations with those who were not there.

Brian was watching football in the front room with the sound down low for Sara's sake. Sara was cooking with Emma in the kitchen and watching Emily play with Peter and her "friends." Brian observed Emily for a moment and then turned his attention back to the game.

"*Strange kid,*" he thought.

Sara finally said, "She'll continue to talk with spirits until someone convinces her they don't exist. Let's not tell Brian what's going on. I'd rather he not say anything to Emily."

"I agree." Emma nodded as she took the spaghetti off the stove and poured out the hot water.

Peter knew better than to argue with Sara when it came to this topic. Neither did he argue with Emma. He believed she and Sara had something which bonded them together, even though he didn't agree with all of it. He was certain there was something "over there," but he didn't really want to know. He was afraid the more he knew, the closer to death he would be. Better to just stay ignorant and leave things to the experts, those being Sara and Emma and now Emily.

And it seemed the more Emily grew the more she would talk to those only she could see. She had conversations in her own language which would go on for what seemed like hours. She played by herself, talking to her dolls and toys and setting up scenarios for herself and her unseen friends.

When Peter would sit with her she would engage him in the play. He was beginning to understand most of everything she was talking about, and who she thought she was talking too. After a while he realized there was someone named Yesh or Josh. Emily's speech was still a little rough, but there was also someone named Terta or Kerra. They seemed to instigate the play time and Emily would respond to questions about who Peter was.

"He Papa." A long pause. "No, he lives at Grammy house but stay here too. He plays toys with me."

"Who are you talking to Em?" Peter asked.

"Terra silly," Emily responded. "She like you Papa."

"Well, I like her too."

Emily loved to play with all the Unseen. She learned so much from them and they were kind and gentle with her. They helped her with her speech and her creativity. Emma knew there was someone with her, but wasn't sure exactly what was going on. She didn't want to interfere but kept a watchful eye during playtime. When Emily asked her to play she stopped everything to participate

Chapter 3

It was early November, and the beginning of winter for Sara. The autumn evenings were finally growing colder, and the leaves were turning. As far as Sara was concerned winter wouldn't be far behind. Most would say winter in Phoenix wasn't winter at all, but those who grew up there had their jackets and boots ready. She always said it wouldn't cool off from the summer swelter until the end of October. Somehow she and Peter made it through another grueling hot summer, thankful for the little cabin they rented every year in Flagstaff. They had been retired now for several years and could come and go as they pleased.

The cabin gave them peace. The only telephones available were their cell phones, no internet, or television. Sara loved to read, and writing was her passion. Peter's passion was woodworking with small tools, this time creating a little town with miniature buildings, streets, cars, and animals. It took incredible patience and Sara would marvel at how beautiful his work was.

Peter had not been feeling well for weeks and he could hide it for only so long. Running to the bathroom every time they sat down for a meal didn't help either. He acted like everything was fine, but Sara knew better.

"Why don't' you go to the doctor instead of throwing up all the time?" Sara finally asked, annoyed.

"There's nothing really wrong. I've just go the flu," he looked away. A dead giveaway he was lying.

"With the flu you have a fever and you are sick for a few days. You don't have a fever and I know you've been sick for at least two weeks. Now do I have to make the appointment for you or are you going to?" she asked in a harsh tone.

Sara had suspected for weeks now that something was wrong with Peter. One day at the cabin he had been walking around the house without his shirt and she saw a lump on his chest.

"What's that?" she asked as she placed her hand over it. An overwhelming feeling of dread hit her in her heart and her stomach. She felt sick and dizzy all at the same time.

"Oh God, no," she said quietly, almost to herself.

"Oh, it's nothing. Just a bump. It was bigger before but now it's smaller, and it feels like it's moving around. It can't be anything bad if it's moving, right?" He tried not to look at her. The last thing he wanted to talk about was this lump and his constant nausea.

She removed her hand from his chest. "You're going to call tomorrow or I am. The kids can only take care of the pets for so long. We are leaving tomorrow anyway."

Sometimes Sara hated her intuition. The reality of Peter's illness was creeping in on her. She closed her eyes and took a few deep breaths.

"I can get through this," she thought. *"We can get through this."*

They spent the next day packing the few things they had brought with them, loading the truck with pine cones and stones Sara had collected. Peter put his miniature town in a box for safety, thinking Emily would love playing with it.

They drove to Phoenix mostly in silence. Sara knew their peace was over as they left the mountain. It was time to take up arms as they say, time to start a battle no one knew if Peter would win or not. When they arrived, Peter unpacked the truck and Sara went inside to call the doctor. She was not going to allow Peter to go another day without being seen. As luck would have it, the office had a late afternoon appointment the following day.

Dr. Peggy Sanders had been the one to first see Peter. She was tall and slim, in her 40s with medium length brown hair and brown eyes. She had a wonderful bed-side manner, always joking with her patients, having them participate in their health-care decisions, instead of dictating what they were going to do.

"OK, Peter. Let's see where you are."

Dr. Sanders did the typical exam, listening to Peter's heart and breathing, checking his blood pressure, ears and eyes. Sara was seated in the back of the room, watching every move. When she had Peter lay down, Sara stood and came over to the table.

"Right there, Doctor." Sara pointed to the area where she had felt the lump. "He's lost a lot of weight lately too and can't keep anything down."

"I see. Does it hurt when I push on it?" She gently moved her fingers around his chest.

"No Doc, not at all. It just moves." Peter gave the appearance of not being concerned, but Sara could hear it in his voice.

"Alright, you can sit up now. I'm going to order some blood tests and x-rays. I want to rule out anything major. Of course when we see someone losing the amount of weight you have, 15 pounds in fact, in less than 2 months without trying to diet, we really need to rule out some type of cancer. The blood work will help with that. I'm going to send you to a gastroenterologist to take a look too."

"Well I can't argue with two women," Peter joked. In reality fear was beginning to touch him.

Sara was amazed at how quickly the appointment for the next doctor happened. Usually it took weeks to see a specialist. Three days later, after his visit with Dr. Sanders, Peter was at the gastroenterologist, having what he called "a look see" down his esophagus.

The test results from the gastroenterologist were a devastating blow to them, but Sara had expected it for some time now. Peter had cancer of the esophagus. More tests and CT scans showed it had already progressed to his bones and had lodged itself in several of his organs.

Now a new part of their journey together began. A life changing journey affecting not only Sara and Peter, but the rest of their family. Their moments together became more precious. Although they rarely argued, now there was no arguing at all. Each one was looking out for the other.

"After all these years I still stand by you and believe in you, no matter what," Sara began to cry. "I love you always."

"And I love you. You always stood strong with whatever happened. When Emily was in the hospital, you were great. I have no worries. I'll beat whatever comes along. I can do it because of you, and only because of you."

Peter held her close, stroking her hair. Somehow he had to get through this. Maybe now was the time to pray. Maybe now it was alright to talk to God about it.

"Hey God, I know it's been a while, but are you still there? I haven't talked to you other than to cuss, and say things like, 'what now, God?' But if you don't mind, I think I'd like to have a conversation."

Peter sat quietly in a little chapel at the Monastery he had been introduced to a long time ago. He decided to take a drive by himself on the Saturday before his Monday appointment with the oncologist. Some friends of his were members of this church and firmly believed in whatever the Bible said. Often they would invite Sara and Peter to come with them, but both had declined, saying it wasn't really for them. Now, desperate for an answer, Peter decided to take a drive and see if he could find what he was missing.

"I just don't understand how this can happen so fast," he said, talking quietly in the chapel. "Tell me why, God. Please tell me where you've been during all of this. I don't want to die, but most of all I don't want to leave Sara and the kids."

The silence of the chapel he had chosen to sit in was beautiful. The Monastery was several miles out of town and consisted of one large Chapel and several smaller ones. He couldn't hear any outside noise but could hear some faint ringing in his ears. As he gazed around from his seat in the back, he could see the Alter adorned with gold and silver icons. Behind the Alter was a huge stained glass with an image of multiple angels looking up.

He followed the gaze of the Angels to see an incredible mural, one of Jesus holding out his hands to his sides, a crown of gold with carvings and impressions Peter couldn't identify and dressed in a gown of gold and blue. The walls of the chapel seemed to surround him with peaceful light dancing off of the stained glass. The rows of seats were hard wood, covered in a dark lacquer. Peter breathed in the Peace that was in the room.

Peter longed for a response to his one-sided conversation but didn't seem to hear anything. After a while, he walked out of the chapel, instinctively placing his hand on his chest, where one of the now many lumps had been growing. He moved his hand from side to side, searching for the lump, but he couldn't find it. It was gone. It had completely disappeared. In fact, all of them were gone.

"I should have been talking to you all along I guess. Thank you for not leaving me," Peter spoke with all humility. Silently, with tears in his eyes, he got back in his car and drove home.

Chapter 4

It was a Monday afternoon and Dr. Marcus Donaldson had taken Peter's appointment quickly. The findings were grim. Dr. Donaldson's stoic demeanor surprised Peter and Sara. They had expected a more personable man. He was in his early 60s, and what hair he had left was gray. His build was big and stocky, too much weight around his middle and the weight of the world on his shoulders.

"You have a very aggressive form of esophageal cancer. The tumor is at the base, where your esophagus meets your stomach. That's why you've not been able to keep anything down. It's too large to operate and you are in no condition to withstand the operation. The biggest problem is, it has spread throughout your body. If it were just in the esophagus, we would do the surgery. But it's in most of your bones and in your lungs. This has been progressing for a long time."

Peter sat dumbfounded. He knew it was bad, but didn't have a clue it was this bad. All Dr. Donaldson had done was to confirm what Sara already knew. Her intuition had told her months before he was ill, but she hadn't wanted to acknowledge it. She decided to put a look of toughness on her face, one that would remain for the next year. Sara had noticed a ringing in her ears a few weeks earlier, but now it intensified. This only irritated her and distracted her from what the doctor was saying.

"So, are you saying I'm done here?" Peter asked with a little sarcastic laugh.

"I'm saying you are terminal. You have maybe less than a year."

Dr. Donaldson was not known for giving any news softly. He was hardcore, right to the point at all times. Saying it any other way didn't make it any easier to take so, in his mind, being direct was the best way.

Remembering his visit to the Monastery, Peter sat up straight and frowned.

"I'm not going to give up. I can make it a lot longer than that. What kind of treatment is there?" He felt he was already on his way to recovery.

"Well, there is the conventional chemotherapy. It will shrink the tumor in your esophagus and those in your bones for the time being. But this is aggressive, and if it spreads any more than it has, then there is not much else we can do. Radiation is also an option but I want to start the chemo first."

Dr. Donaldson never looked at Peter or Sara. He sat at his desk with his head down and thumbed through the papers in front of him, writing illegible notes on some of the pages.

"Ok, so when do we start?" Peter's tone became one of determination and he was ready to do battle.

"Let's talk with scheduling. I'll have one of the case managers speak to you about the way this works." He quickly stood up and left the room, leaving Peter and Sara with the news.

"I'm not giving up, you know. I've got too much to do still." He said with confidence. He took her hand in his and looked directly into her eyes.

Sara sat quietly, not wanting to speak or move. She knew of the war Peter was about to go into and it would not be easy for him, or for the family. She had seen friends die of this horrible disease called cancer. There were alternative forms of treatment she wanted to talk with him about, but she hesitated.

"And I don't want any of your woowoo stuff either. I want to do whatever the doctor says," Peter insisted, almost reading her mind.

Sara was saddened by his decision, but not surprised. He had always tolerated what he called her "woowoo" beliefs. She was of a more metaphysical or new age philosophy. Even though she had joined the Lutheran church, she had always believed there was more to life than what she was taught.

Sara's church was now her garden, being outside in nature, and talking to God. She listened to music that moved her and talked to God every day, thanking for him for the beautiful life she had. But she couldn't resist the services led by Pastor Paul, the lovely music and the socialization, so she attended Sunday services as well.

"You will have whatever you want, Pete," gently squeezing his hand. "This is your body, your journey and I will support whatever decision you make. If you don't want treatment then I will support you."

"What do you mean if I don't want treatment? I want to fight this thing. I can do it with chemo and radiation and that's what I'm going to do." Peter was angry, not with Sara, but with the fact that he had been given such grim news.

The door opened and Russ, their case manager, walked in. He was a big guy, about 6'1", balding, overweight and dressed in his hospital greens. "Why don't you guys follow me?" he said with a smile.

Russ left the room and Peter and Sara followed. They walked past a nurse's station and into a large room with 12 reclining chairs arranged in the shape of a large rectangle. Eight of them were filled with people who were hooked to IV lines and receiving some kind of treatment.

"Over here," Russ motioned.

They went into a side room where he had Peter sit in a small chair. "I'm your resident vampire. I'm going to take your blood, get your vitals and hand you a bunch of brochures you're never going to read. Now pull up your sleeve and we'll get started, big guy."

Russ's demeanor was completely opposite of Dr. Donaldson. He was jovial and always had a smile on his face. Peter did as he was told as Sara took the brochures from Russ and sat just outside the room. He was right, she would never read these. Her eyes were blurry as she looked at them. She glanced around the room, at the faces of those who were sitting in the chairs receiving treatment. A few nurses were moving from one person to another, checking their IV lines, asking questions and speaking quietly. As Sara looked out the big picture window on the opposite side of the room, she could see the tall skyscrapers in the distance, ones she had worked in while she was employed.

Over the next few weeks, the clinic hired more nurses. It seemed cancer had become an epidemic. What they didn't know was history had begun to repeat itself. It was a plague no one wanted to talk about. There were fundraisers, laboratories, hospitals, clinics, but no one was getting a handle on it. The statistics were mind boggling on the chances of getting some kind of cancer. To Sara, this seemed like big business. It was the unspoken pandemic no one wanted to face.

Peter began his treatments the following Friday. The Wednesday before, he went for outpatient surgery to have a shunt implanted so they could pump chemotherapy directly into his veins. He was to have chemotherapy all day on Friday and take a pump home with him that would administer the chemo for the next few days. Then on Monday he would return and Russ would take the pump off.

Being diagnosed with this life-threatening disease caused him to rethink his position on God and reminded him of his time at the Monastery. He observed the others around him; their expressions of pain, worry, concern and fear; the hope and the sadness. He prayed they would be alright and have the strength to get through this. He felt comfortable in the knowledge he would be fine and what he was doing was right. His belief is what kept him going and he was healing. Peter believed God was guiding the doctors and nurses and he was getting what he needed. He had convinced himself he would be alright. At least for now.

He could feel the pain of those around him; especially the young ones. When Peter looked in their eyes, he saw fear and hopelessness and it hurt. By observing them, he began to feel what they felt and it overwhelmed him. When this would happen, he would pray. Pray for them to find to find peace, strength, to be able to endure.

The young ones were very reluctant to talk. They wanted to know why they were there with all these old people dying. The others would talk about what they were going through, the types of cancer, how long it had been and the outcomes. Some had the same type of cancer, while others had a different form. But cancer is cancer.

Some people would get blood transfusions along with chemo. Those in their 60s and older had positive attitudes. But you could always tell who the first timer's were. They were concerned, wondering what would happen to them. The people working there had their hearts in the right place. They were attentive and caring without being full of pity. Each of them made the patients feel they were human beings and not the disease which had engulfed them.

Peter had a lot of positive feelings while at the clinic, but much sadness too. It was obvious some patients would not return. For the staff, there were no rich or poor, no gender or race. The patents were all the same. All were there for the same reasons. Those who wanted to survive no matter what and those who just wanted the pain to go away.

Peter began to pray for the people who worked there. It had to be hard to see those who wouldn't return. He sometimes felt there was more he should do, but wasn't sure how to approach it. He prayed for God to comfort them and help them get through the bad part of the treatments. If they could just accept what would happen in the next few days and how hard it was going to be; to just look toward the end of the week, then it would be alright.

He would speak to one person and others would listen and join the conversation. Some would ask questions, and he hoped he was guided to give them God's answers, not his own. He prayed they would feel what he felt, that it was going to be alright and he would heal. And if he didn't, then it was his time to go. He prayed they would accept God in their heart as he had, just a short time ago at the Monastery. He finally came to the conclusion no more could be done; they just needed to have faith.

There was so much need in the treatment room. He could feel most of the patients didn't want to ask for help believing it was easier to keep this very private. He just wanted to go over to them, wrap his arms around them and say, "It's Okay." But what bothered him most about being there was the cumulative fear of no tomorrow.

It seemed the other patients had to understand tomorrow was not a promise, it was a gift and they could only live for today. For Peter, it was the most important thing to remember. To give as much of themselves today and it would come back tenfold. To let the anger go, to stop being afraid no matter how hard. Once they learned there was nothing to fear it was easy. Then he would start to observe them and feel the fear going around the room. He would just pray harder, believing God would ease it by the end of the day. This was the experience Peter needed; to know God was with him.

Peter would get overwhelmed when he spoke of God now. As he would pray he would find peace to help him get over the erratic emotions. The chemo and other drugs made him emotional. He knew it was alright to show emotion, but it was hard to talk to someone when he couldn't stop crying. But now it was a release of the emotions and it was not something he could control any longer. He had been good at controlling his emotions all his life but now it was almost impossible. The release was there and he had to accept it.

He knew there were going to be bad days after the treatment but with each treatment, his chances of living increased. The people who worked there had such a positive attitude, it reinforced his as well. Observing how they dealt with the treatments and people all day; their ability to focus and express compassion at such a strong level, made it obvious they were chosen for this purpose. Peter believed God put them in this clinic to help those who couldn't help themselves.

Chapter 5

PETER HAD BEEN IN AND out of the hospital many times during his treatments. In preparation for his chemo treatments, Peter went as an outpatient to the hospital for a port-a-cath. A small IV line placed under the skin in his chest. This allowed the doctors and nurses direct access to his blood to give him chemo and generally treat him without having to stick him every time. After his treatments began to make him sick, he had surgery for a feeding tube. Eating had become almost impossible. He couldn't keep anything down and he was losing weight rapidly. The tube placement was easy, like the placement of the port, and he was in and out of surgery in a few hours.

Sara drove him to get the feeding tube and sat in the cafeteria waiting for him. She brought a book but couldn't remember anything she read. Her mind was on the possible future. A future without Peter.

This is just not happening! She thought.

Although her denial was huge, reality had hit her long ago. She found eating difficult as well. No feeding tube for her. Forcing everything was the key. Forcing to stay positive, forcing the lightness in her voice, forcing the smiles. It wasn't too difficult because Peter had such a good outlook on everything. He always had.

But this was different. They had never experienced anything like this. While she had vague memories of being a caretaker, possibly in another life, none of it seemed real. She had what she called visions of another time, when she had lost a son and a best friend. The hospitalizations, the assisting with the medications, this all seemed so familiar, yet not. What was this about?

Peter's first treatment was brutal. He came home from spending all day at the clinic and went straight to bed. Sara was relieved because she was alone to cry silently in the other room. After a few hours she went in to check on him.

"Peter, are you awake?" She moved around to the side of the bed.

He moaned and turned toward her. He had been lying on his side. The wound from the port was fresh and the bandages needed to be changed.

"Peter, I have to change your bandage. Can you hold still for me?"

"Yes. I feel horrible. I think I'm going to be sick!"

Peter got up and sprinted to the bathroom, his pants nearly falling to his knees. His t-shirt hung on him, his muscular frame slowly deteriorating. She could hear him losing what little he had in his stomach. He couldn't afford to drop any more weight and it was so distressing to her as she sat on the edge of the bed, waiting for him to come out. She had brought all the supplies to clean his wound and was ready for when he came back. He staggered out of the bathroom, holding onto the frame.

"I want to go outside. I want a cigarette."

"OK, I'll go with you after we change your dressing."

She had always hated his smoking but she was not going to ask him to quit now. They walked together out to the back yard. Peter had worked so hard on the yard and created a beautiful place for them. The trees were a luscious dark green, and the flowers were of all different colors in pots surrounding the yard. He had made a sanctuary for them. They sat at the table surrounded by the sweet smells of the flowers and sounds of doves cooing in the trees.

"I'm not going to pick on you for smoking, but it would be better for you if you stopped. I'm not suggesting now but soon, when you are stronger. Maybe you could cut back a little."

Peter spoke softly, "I've thought about it, but what's the point in stopping now? I'm not going to die from smoking. Besides, I'm dead anyway."

"What?' Sara was completely taken by surprise. "What happened to 'I'm going to fight this, I'm going to show you I'm not a statistic and I'll live long after everyone thought I would die'?" The stress in her voice was obvious to her and Peter.

"You just don't know, I could go tomorrow and smoking gives me pleasure. I can't eat anything anyway. By the way, when are the kids coming? I need to talk to my Dad and tell him that I can't work in the garage this weekend."

Sara had been facing the flower garden, sitting next to Peter. A cool breeze swept over her, ever so slightly moving her hair, as she turned her head to the side to look at him. What was he saying? The kids were all out of town. She had told him so when they got home from the clinic and his dad had passed away 15 years ago.

"Peter, are you alright?"

"What?" Peter hung his head and took a long drag off his cigarette.

"I said, are you alright? You said you can't work in your Dad's garage this weekend." Sara tried to keep her voice still in spite of the rising panic she was feeling.

"Well he's going to be pretty mad at me if I don't show up!" Peter was beginning to look and sound very confused.

"OK. I think we need to take a ride to the hospital." Sara got up from her chair. "Let's put out the cigarette and get in the car."

"Whatever you say Mom. You always know what's best." He put his cigarette out and stood on wobbly legs. She helped him put on his shoes and struggled to get him in the car.

The chemo had been too strong for him. He was beginning to lose his mind and he was very weak. Traffic was light but people were driving aggressively, which made Sara even more distressed. Peter sat quietly during the ride, mumbling something about being late for school, not getting his homework done and dad would be mad at him.

Peter slowly got out of the car and into the wheelchair Sara had found just inside the door. It was flu season and the emergency room was a mess. She wheeled him to the desk.

"My husband has cancer. He's having hallucinations and needs to see a doctor right away. He came home from a chemo treatment earlier this afternoon and he's very sick."

The emergency room had become a dumping ground for the sick. If they didn't have health insurance, doctors would not see them. Legally, the hospital could not turn anyone away. So few could afford health insurance which made their only resource was the ER. They would deal with the bill some other time. Sara estimated 40 people occupying all the available chairs.

"Alright, let's get his info. Has he been here before?" The attendant was obviously irritated at another person coming through his doors.

"Yes, he's Peter Hansen," Sara quickly replied. The attendant entered his name in the computer where all of his personal information came up immediately. He verified with Sara he had the right Peter Hansen, printed out wrist band, placed it on Peter and instructed them to take a seat, if they could find one.

Sara wheeled Peter to the doorway of the nearest hall. He was leaning on his elbow, head in hand, eyes closed. She leaned against the wall behind him, anxiously listening to every name called before them.

After 10 minutes, Peter's name was called. Sara was so relieved, since she had counted so many people in the waiting room. The nurse began taking his vitals and entering them in the computer. She barely looked at Peter and Sara became very annoyed. It was beginning to feel like Peter wasn't a priority, in fact wasn't important at all.

"Alright Mr. Hansen, go take a seat. Someone will call you when it's your turn," the uncaring nurse motioned towards the waiting room and dismissed them as if they didn't even exist.

After the first two hours, with Peter sleeping uncomfortably in the wheelchair, talking on and off to his mom and dad, Sara went to the desk to ask how long they anticipated the wait would be. The how long question would arise five more times in the next three hours until she began to yell at the staff.

"Sara, would you let Buster outside? He keeps licking my hand and barking. Can't you hear him?"

"That's it!" Sara got out of the chair she was able to snag two hours ago and marched to the registration desk.

"I want you to call an ambulance," She stood in front of the registration nurse with her arms crossed. "I want an ambulance to take him to another hospital right now!"

"Mrs. Hansen, all the hospitals are having the same problem we are having. A few have closed their emergency rooms and are redirecting people here. There's nothing we can do about it," the nurse spoke, with only irritation in her voice and little compassion. "You'll just have to wait."

"That's no longer an option! These people behind us have a paper cut!" Sara gestured with a wide sweeping motion of her right arm. "My husband is hallucinating and almost falling out of the chair he's in. We've been here five hours now. I've seen people go back there who came in 15 minutes ago. What the hell is that about?"

"Mrs. Hansen, we have to take people as they come in and evaluate their situation. If it is minor then we treat them right away in an area designed for their situation and get them moving along. If it's more complicated, there is a specific area in the hospital designed to take care of them. Your husband is one of those more complicated patients and we are waiting for a space for him."

"Unacceptable. Unacceptable! Someone needs to look at him now, and I'm not going to listen to any more bullshit," she said very matter of factly.

"Alright, bring him here and we'll take a look." The nurse rolled her eyes at the others sitting beside her.

Sara had been very loud, loud enough so everyone in the room heard her, including the patients she had just gestured to. She didn't care. She was trying to take care of her husband and all of her frustration over the last few months had came tumbling out of her. She retrieved Peter from his position next to the hallway and wheeled him to the desk.

"So what's going on Mr. Hansen?" The nurse placed all her attention on Peter.

"I don't know. May be too much chemo I guess." Peter had come back mentally for a moment but his appearance said otherwise.

"Alright. We'll call you as soon as we can." She turned away from Peter, preparing for the next triage patient.

"What is going on? He thinks he's at home! He just asked me what's for dinner and when is his program on. He's talking about our dog that died years ago. You've made us sit here for hours. I want you to call an ambulance and get him to another facility. I don't care if its flu season or not. He's not supposed to be around sick people either and you've got us sitting out there in the middle of all that coughing and sneezing. They need a band aid, he needs a doctor! He's having a bad reaction to his chemo and is in distress. Get him back there now!"

Her protests were ignored by the nurses, but not by the security guard who was coming down the hallway. She decided she needed to soften up a bit. This guy looked like trouble. "Can we at least have a mask for him?" Sara asked, with a slightly toned down voice.

"Sure." The nurse handed Sara a mask and went back to her paperwork.

"Here honey, put this on." Sara reached around Peter's head and placed the mask over his nose and mouth.

"I look pretty silly Mom," he looked up smiling at her.

"See!" Sara said loudly as she looked back at the nurse. "He just called me Mom!"

"OK, OK, I see," she snapped. Obviously the day had gotten to her as well. It was impossible to please everyone and to this nurse Peter wasn't in any obvious distress. She stood, walking away from them, getting the next chart and calling a name.

The nurse's attempt to calm her down was pointless. She had lost all sense of politeness. Sara decided if she made enough of a ruckus, they would respond and it worked. A nurse Sara had never seen went to Peter and re-checked his vitals and it was obvious he was slipping.

"There must have been a shift change," Sara said to the new nurse. "I bet they told you to watch out for me." The nurse smiled at Sara knowingly telling them it would be no more than five minutes. Another 15 minutes went by before she returned to collect Peter and Sara into a room in the back.

This was the first of many hospital stays during Peter's chemotherapy treatment. The doctors adjusted his medications so that he was not so overwhelmed when he had a treatment and he improved. At one point, Peter went into remission after a few months, but it didn't last. The cancer had come back with a vengeance, as cancer always does.

It's a sneaky disease, hiding in places the doctors couldn't see and didn't know where to look. It fed on sugar and stress. The more sugar Peter ingested, the more the cancer was fed until it became so large it had to show itself. Sara called Peter a sugaraholic. He would eat large candy bars in one sitting while watching a movie or The Weather Channel. He loved the weather and since most of his family lived elsewhere, he could watch what was going on back home. A large candy bar would be gone without him even noticing and the weight never piled on him. If Sara looked at a candy bar she would gain a pound, and if she ate one she would gain two.

By now Sara struggled with trying to get Peter to eat. With her being Italian eating was a part of life. But Peter's appetite was gone and he was beginning to refuse her offers. One day while running errands, she called him at the hospital to check in. She had gone home the night before, frustrated at his refusal to eat much that day.

"Peter, I've decided I'm not going to harass you any more about eating. It's just too frustrating for me. I get all worked up about your nutrition and you obviously don't care. So if you want to eat, eat. If you don't, then don't. I'm not going to say anything about it anymore." She had tried to be gentle but frustration was coming out in her tone.

"Are you giving up?" he asked timidly.

"No, I'm not but I think you are. I think you need to eat and the doctors think you need to eat."

Peter had the feeding tube removed a few months prior because it was irritating his stomach and causing him a lot of pain. He had promised Doc. Donaldson he would maintain his weight and nutrition but he was no longer capable of keeping this promise.

"Well I'm not giving up!" he said defiantly. "When are you coming?"

She told him she would arrive shortly, ending the conversation with an "I love you". Concluding her errands, she drove robotically to the hospital. When she arrived at his room, he had a wheelchair waiting for him.

"I want to go to the cafeteria," he said with a smile.

"Great!" she helped him into the chair.

Peter had the nurses unhook him from the IV lines and he was ready to go. He had taken her comments as a challenge; one he would not regret. Nothing appealed to him at the cafeteria, but he picked out some fruit and toast, taking them back to his room and gagged them down.

He wanted to please Sara, at all costs, because he loved her so much. He was so overwhelmed with this illness and what it was doing to her and the kids. He saw her sadness, heartache, even though she had tried to stifle it. They had been together too long for her to be able to hide much. Yet she tried and he knew why. He understood she was just trying to be strong for him. And he wanted to be strong for her in return. It was impossible for him to explain how eating was more than a chore, it was almost impossible. Everything about food repulsed him. How do you explain that? It was an overwhelming challenge, and even though he liked challenges, sometimes he couldn't face it. Yet he would try for Sara. He would try for her peace of mind.

Chapter 6

Music defined Sara and for the last few days she had a song in her head that would not go away. It was about the last days of two people, where one would die and the other would have to stay behind. The songwriter wanted to stay awake, because if he fell asleep, she might be gone. It was very fitting for what was happening with her now. She had gone to the hospital to see Peter and on this particular day, Sara felt he was slipping away. He had curled up in the bed in a fetal position, and slept very hard. The bed was at an angle where he had folded himself up in the middle. She walked in to see him trying to sit upright, using the controls to move the feet down and head up on the bed.

"Sara," he said holding his hand out to her. She walked around the bed, took his hand and sat in the chair by him.

"When I fell asleep I went to this place," he continued. "It was a beautiful meadow with dark green trees, and a bright light. There was no pain and more peace than I have ever experienced. I was standing on the edge and all I had to do was step in and I would be gone from here. I've been to the meadow twice now. Each time I said, 'No, not now.' But I know all I had to do was walk in and everything would change. Everything would be fine."

"Was there anyone waiting for you? Did you see anyone?" Sara asked quietly, gently stroking his hand, while she looked deeply in his eyes.

"No, I didn't see anyone. Just this beautiful meadow." he explained. "There were wild flowers surrounded by tall aspen trees."

"Then it's not your time honey. When you go to the meadow and it's your time, you will see someone. Someone will be there to greet you. I'm sure of it."

This was a huge sign to Sara and she knew his time was near. She brought him home a few days later. There was nothing else the doctors could do for him at this time, and he was stable. One night soon after they were in bed, Peter was sleeping and she was not. She was watching him reach out, as though he was trying to grasp something. It was another sign to her and she began to prepare herself and their children. She had talked to Brian and Emma about the dying process; it was coming and they needed to be prepared too. It was part of life and it couldn't be stopped, no matter what they did or how hard they tried. Peter's time on earth was about to come to an end.

Sara quietly sang the song in her head trying to stay awake, repeating it to help her cope. Tears streamed down her face as she watched her beloved begin to cross over.

The last hospital visit was brutal. She had noticed Peter was not sure what time of the day it was or if she had been there or not. Sara mentioned this to his doctors and they decided to do an MRI. The results were bad; the cancer had spread to his brain. The report showed new spots on his brain and the results indicated there was nothing they could do. He was too weak to withstand any more treatments. The doctors and Sara decided to bring him home.

By now Peter was in a wheelchair most of the time. He could walk short distances around the house, but to go anywhere other than room to room, he needed the chair. He had always resisted getting a handicapped parking sticker, but Brian had insisted and had taken Sara to MVD to get one. Dr. Donaldson had given them the necessary paperwork, and now Peter was glad they had taken the time. Brian would help get the wheelchair out of the trunk of the car and place his dad in it whenever they had to be somewhere.

A few days after his last hospital stay, Brian and Sara brought Peter to see his primary care doctor. He was not scheduled for any more chemo treatments, but Dr. Sanders wanted to take a look at him. It had been a little more than a year since he had seen Peter. He had passed the one year mark he had vowed to make by one month. While Dr. Donaldson had kept Doc. Sanders up to date on Peter's condition, she had a feeling it would help if she saw him for routine care.

Peter and Sara did not have to wait long once they arrived. The nurse came to get him, smiling and kneeled beside him, taking his hand. She gave him a hug and directed them to a room down the hall. Soon Dr. Sanders came into the room, sat on the chair and looked at her chart. It was obvious to her what Peter's condition was. He was frail, weighing only 102 pounds, his hair was mostly gone, and his color gray. His head was bowed in the wheelchair and he struggled to stay awake.

"Good afternoon everybody." She glanced wisely at Sara and Brian, then at Peter.

"Hi Doc. How's it going for you?" Peter asked, bending forward, looking at his lap.

"I'm very well as usual. Let's take a look at you." She put her stethoscope into her ears and wheeled close to him. She listened to his heart, took his blood pressure and temperature. She was always hands-on with him and treated him with great respect. As she wrote in her chart she looked at Peter.

"Well, what are we going to do with you mister?" she asked with concern in her voice.

"Not a whole lot! I'm just fine. A little tired, but I'm doing great." Peter didn't look at her, but kept his head bowed.

"Any pain?" she asked.

"Oh yes, always. But it comes with the territory," he murmured, still not looking up from his lap.

"How about we make a call to Hospice? They can help manage your pain better," she suggested.

"Oh no, I don't need those guys. I'm just fine without them." Peter had felt Hospice was a sign of weakness; a sign of death's door just around the corner.

Dr. Sanders glanced at Sara. She nodded her head, knowing this was the next step and Dr. Sanders nodded back.

"Okay then. How about if I get you another prescription for some pain meds and I see you in a few weeks?" She grabbed her prescription pad out of the pocket of her white coat and began writing on the countertop.

"That's okay with me. I've got my drivers here, so I can be on all the pain meds I want. Brian is the heavy lifter and Sara is the co-pilot," he joked.

Dr. Sanders said her goodbyes and left the room. As Brian wheeled Peter out to the car, Sara gathered the prescriptions. One was for Vicodin and the other was for Hospice.

"I think you'll need this to have them come. They usually need authorization from one of us. Paper work you know," Dr. Sanders was referring to the prescription for Hospice. "He doesn't have long."

"I know. Thank you for taking care of him," Sara spoke, with tears in her eyes. She was glad Brian had taken him to the car.

"Is there anything I can do for you?" Dr. Sanders asked.

"No. My kids are helping with everything. I'm so blessed by them. I don't know what I'd do if they weren't there for us." Sara turned and left quietly before the tears fell.

Sara knew she was going to have to make the call. Brian had work and Emma had Emily to take care of. Tom was in Afghanistan and she didn't want to burden Emma any more than she already had. They were available to help, but she also wanted them to be able to tend to their own lives.

She made the call to Hospice when they got home. Brian took Peter into the bedroom and got him settled in while she was on the phone. She felt it was better Peter not hear her phone conversation. This particular Hospice organization was non-profit, but they did accept insurance if it was available along with donations. A nurse was scheduled to visit that evening to evaluate Peter. Pleased at how quickly they responded and how compassionate they were on the phone, Sara knew she made the right choice.

Once Peter was comfortable, Brian left for the pharmacy to pick up the prescription and stopped by the grocery store to grab some dinner. He wanted to be at the house when the nurse came, but he also wanted his parents to have some time alone too. He called Emma to tell her what the doctor had said.

"I'm going to come over and bring Emily. She will cheer them both up," Emma cried softly as she spoke to Brian.

She had tears in her voice, but pushed them down so no one would know. The tears would return when she was safely alone, either in the car or in the shower. Those were the best places to cry where no one would see. Her best conversations with God were in these places.

"Good idea, Sis. I'll be there right after I finish at the store. Have Emily save her appetite. Somehow I don't think Dad's going to eat." Brian hung up and grabbed a few extra things, anticipating his mom hadn't been to the grocery store in a while.

Peter had given up food. It was so difficult to swallow and his stomach always protested. Brian picked up Peter's favorite chicken and side dishes and returned to their house, hoping he would try a little bit. If he and Sara ate some, then maybe Peter would be encouraged to. Brian's fear was he was losing his Dad and his Mom wouldn't make it without her beloved husband. He knew she was strong willed, but she loved Peter so much the thought of him being gone might be too much for her. When Brian returned, she was sitting in her chair at the kitchen table.

"I'm back Mom," Brian yelled from the front door.

"I'm in here." It was nearly a whisper filled with despair. Brian brought the food in and placed the bags on the table. Sara stood and hugged him, crying ever so slightly.

"I've known for a few days something was happening." She sat back down, slumping in her chair. "He's been reaching out for something while we're in bed at night. I can't see what he's reaching for, but it's like he's grabbing at something and being pulled, ever so gently, from the room."

"I don't understand. What do you mean?" Brian was visibly confused.

Sara hung her head as she spoke. "I mean I think 'they' are trying to help him over. He had told me about a time during his last hospital stay while he was sleeping he saw a meadow of some sort. He was standing on the edge and felt if he just stepped inside it, he would be gone from here. This happened to him twice, but there was no one to greet him, so I'm sure he wasn't ready. Now, I think he is seeing someone and they are reaching out for him. Either that, or sometimes it looks like he's pushing away a curtain and looking into a room. He reaches out more than he pushes."

"I'm not sure what's happening, other than maybe a vivid dream Mom" Brian was trying to rationalize the irrational.

"But every night? And the same dream? I don't think so. I believe he's seeing the other side. I've heard about it. Just before my friend Sandy's husband died he did the same thing, or at least something like it."

Hospice had a booklet they gave to her friend Sandy and it talked about the stages of dying. This was one of them Sara had remembered. It was important to her that Peter had someone waiting for him. He had been so strong and was always the one who took care of everything. He deserved to not be alone when he died. It made sense to her for someone to be waiting there. In all the stories she had read and the research she had done, people who were about to die all talked about deceased relatives and friends waiting for them.

Sara had an Aunt June who she just adored. A few years before she passed away, she would talk about her deceased brother and sister standing in the doorway of her bedroom, asking her to come with them. Everyone but Sara told her she was getting senile, but Sara believed her.

Brian was beginning to worry about his Mom. She was saying weird stuff and talking to herself a lot lately. She couldn't find the names of things when she was trying to tell him something and he caught her staring at the remote for the TV wondering what it was. At first he thought she was under a lot of stress and she now was paying the price. But with this very strange story he was more concerned about her.

"*What's she talking about?*' he thought to himself. "*I think she may be losing it, plus she's forgetting everything. She couldn't remember where the keys were and I found them in the office. They never put them there. And she hasn't paid any bills for weeks.*"

He made a mental note to talk to Emma about this. As he did, Emma and Emily rang the bell. Sara went to answer as Brian put out the food on the table.

Emily squealed with delight as she saw what was for dinner. "I'm so hungry! I want this, and that and that and that!" she squealed.

"Settle down little one!" Emma always corrected her with love and compassion, but her nerves were worn thin as well.

Sara looked at everyone. "Come on now let's have our last meal together. Brian, go get your Dad."

Chapter 7

THE HOSPICE NURSE CAME TO the door with her black bag and clipboard. Bonnie was a large woman in her 50s with long gray hair braided behind her. To look at her it appeared she was gruff, but her smile gave her away. Brian mused, saying her name should be Helga for Helga's House of Pain. She could tell he was teasing her and made a mental note to give him an especially hard time, jokingly of course. Bonnie visited with Peter for a while in the bedroom, convincing him if he went to a facility for just a few days they could manage his pain better.

"Only if I'm home for Christmas," Peter agreed.

"We'll do everything we can to make that happen," was Bonnie's knowing reply.

A few hours later, after Bonnie had made a couple of calls and Sara filled out some paperwork, a private ambulance came to pick up Peter. Brian took Emily home with him and Emma stayed to drive Sara to the facility. After speeding to keep up with the driver, Sara and Emma finally arrived. Emma was so irritated at him for doing 10 miles over the speed limit, not taking into consideration she didn't know where she was going. Her thought was to complain to the first person she came in contact with. But Sara just took it all in stride, not caring about anything but getting Peter comfortable.

It was a beautiful facility with private rooms and a front desk, almost like an upscale hotel.

"*What a great place,*" Sara thought to herself. "*This will be a good place for Peter to die. And probably a good place for me too.*"

Each room had a large glass arcadia door which opened to a luscious patio with bright flowers, green grass, wind chimes and hummingbird feeders. The only thing that resembled a hospital was the bed. While the rooms were small, the atmosphere was comfortable. The walls were painted a light blue and dotted with white shapes resembling clouds. Two soft, comfortable chairs were stationed on either side of the bed.

It was Wednesday night at 10:30 by the time Peter was settled in. He joked with the nurses about being an old man but they had better watch out for him. They treated him with kindness and respect, making sure all his wants and needs were met. Sara was confident leaving him in their care and asked Emma to take her home.

"I wanted more time," she cried out as she looked up at the ceiling while lying in their bed. "How can you take him away from me? It's just not fair!"

As she lay on her back with eyes closed, and the song about them parting came to her head. While it probably was meant to comfort her, it only succeeded in making her miss him; knowing he would soon be gone.

The next morning Emma brought Emily to the sitter and picked up Sara. They would meet Brian at the Hospice facility later. Emma had put out the word through an email where Peter was. She had included there were no restrictions for visitation and offered everyone a chance to say goodbye. People began to filter in and out the rest of the day. Peter was conscious some of the time, but mostly sleeping. Very close friends of theirs came, or sent messages through email. Everyone supported Peter and the family, offering condolences and assistance.

"This time I'm ready," Peter whispered.

He hadn't spoken since the night before. His eyes were shut and he rested quietly. Sara knew he was standing at the edge of the meadow again.

It had to be what he meant when he said "this time." She, Emma, and Brian were the only people in the room. A nurse walked in to give him some mild pain medication, swabbing the inside of his check and adjusting the covers.

"He said this time he's ready," Sara told her.

"That's very typical. They see something we can't see. They always know there is something else; something besides what is here." She had been a Hospice nurse for 15 years now and had assisted people in their transitions. "It won't be long now."

It was early Friday morning and he lay in his bed, moaning with each breath. The Hospice nurse told them it was called it the death rattle. Sara thought this was a horrible way to refer to it, but she really couldn't come up with anything better. He had been completely unconscious for about 16 hours since his last words. Sara sat next to him on the bed, rubbing his arm. Emily had come to say goodbye and she was in the chair across the room. Brian sat on the other side of the bed holding his dad's hand.

"I don't want Papa to die," Emily said quietly. Emma took her hand, motioned for her to kiss Peter on the cheek. After she did, Emma kissed him too and took Emily from the room.

"Peter, go to the meadow." Sara quietly spoke with a tear in her voice. "Remember? You told me about a meadow that was so beautiful. Look around now. There's someone there waiting for you. You saw the bright light and peacefulness of it, remember? You can stay there as long as you like. It's alright. It's alright now."

As she spoke, his breathing became less restless and the moaning stopped completely. The nurse came in again, giving him some more pain medicine. He opened his eyes for the first time, grasped Sara's hand and looked directly at her. There was no fear. No more pain. She could feel him leave completely. His body took a few more short breaths and he was gone.

Chapter 8

Peter felt the pull. It wasn't a physical pull, but the pull of his soul.

"What is this?" His frown made his eyebrows bend towards his eyes, and the corners of his mouth fell.

"I can't resist it. Wait. I can see some light up ahead. What is that?" He felt confused and his thinking was clouded, along with his vision.

He was standing on a dirt road. Even though it appeared familiar, it wasn't. It weaved slightly towards a large group of towering mountains, but the lighting was dark, it was overcast, and he wasn't able to see clearly.

"Are those people up ahead?"

His head stretched slightly forward, as though his vision might clear. He could see shadows of figures but they were dark too and squinting didn't help. As he stepped forward, the lighting began to get brighter....not enough to see clearly, but a little less cloudy. It was as though someone had their hand on a dimmer switch. With each slow step Peter made, the lighting brightened ever so slightly.

Peter could hear Sara talking behind him, something about a meadow, but it sounded muffled as if she were speaking behind a heavy, thick door. He turned half way around, looking over his shoulder. As he did, the light dimmed again.

"What the heck is happening here?" Peter asked out loud, confused.

He turned back, looking forward again and took a few steps. As he did, the light became brighter than before. With each step the shadows up ahead softened. Peter was now able to see they were people who were moving towards him now; slowly and rhythmically. He began to feel warmth in his heart and a clearing in his head. The light began to get even brighter, although there was no sun that he noticed. There was the feeling of a pull again and this time a gentle push from behind as he began to take a few more steps forward. He could hear people talking behind him but they became more and more distant. He struggled to hear, and struggled to see.

Could it be Sara's voice? It sounded as if she were crying. He turned at the waist to look back and again felt the gentle pull forward. As he felt the pull, he turned forward again. The light became brighter and the figures became more visible. Clearly they were people. Probably ten or maybe fifteen from what he could tell.

Three of them continued to move forward at a faster pace than the others. They didn't really walk; it was more a glide. He could see the others behind them slow down even more as the three began to glow in a sparkling blue-green color emanating all around them.

Now Peter was able to see beautiful green bushes and yellow flowers cascading down the side of a mountain to his left. Saguaro and Cholla cactus dotted the landscape on his right and as he took a deep breath, he could smell mesquite trees. Hills of old volcanic rock were strewn with wild flowers and shrubs farther up to his right. The air was clear and crisp with cool dew. Red bougainvilleas were everywhere. There were no telephone poles or high-powered wires; no billboards, just open space.

"I don't want Papa to die."

It was Emily! Peter turned completely around and the light began to dim.

"I remember that little girl. It's Emily! Emily, I'm here precious. I'm here!" Peter began to panic, not knowing where he was and took a few steps towards Emily's voice in what was becoming darkness again. "I can't see you, where are you?"

Suddenly, the three people who had been coming towards him were surrounding him. Peter became washed with a feeling of love and comfort, surrounded in the soothing blue-green light. He turned to look at them, with sadness on his face and tears in his eyes.

"She will see you, Peter. She has the sight. But first we ask you come with us. There is much to do before you can go back. She will be able to help the others seeing you when you are ready to talk to them."

The Three, as they were referred to by the others, were now clearer but still a little blurry. Peter could make out they were two men and one woman. One was taller than the other two, and had a brighter glow.

The Tall One spoke again. "Peter, my name is Yesh. We've come to walk with you down this road. This is Silas and Tara," he gestured towards the others with a nod of his head.

Peter didn't actually hear words coming from Yesh. It was more of a feeling enveloping him and his mind knew what Yesh was saying. He never felt anything like it before. It took his attention away from Emily. He couldn't stop looking into Yesh's eyes.

Yesh had an air of confidence and incredible peace about him. His hair was dark, his blue eyes were full of love and his voice was deep and soothing. He was dressed in what looked like a robe, but it didn't really have any form and Peter couldn't see his feet. The clothing was a soft green and melted into the already blue-green light which surrounded him. It was impossible to tell his age, but it didn't matter. Peter was amazed by this wonderful man floating in front of him.

Silas was also tall, but a few inches shorter than Yesh. He looked to be in his late 40s with neatly trimmed dark brown hair and brown eyes. He wore jeans and a t-shirt that read "I'm in Heaven." Silas liked to play around, kidding and joking all the time in order to bring smiles to everyone's faces. As Silas smiled at Peter, they made eye contact and Peter immediately knew everything about Silas. Hs playfulness took away Peter's agitation.

Tara was a slim woman in her 30s and had the sweetest smile. Her features were striking with soft flowing blond hair and green eyes. She had the most peaceful expression he had ever seen. She too was glowing and it was difficult to make out what she was wearing. Peter's eyes were still somewhat out of focus. Tara took him by the arm, and gently began to walk down the path and towards the mountains where the others were waiting.

As Peter began to walk forward with Tara, the light began to get brighter. It was then he realized he no longer felt any pain. He looked at his hands; then his feet. Realizing he was dressed in his most comfortable jeans and old ratty t-shirt, he said, "Ah, Sara hates this shirt! But it feels so good, baggy and soft." He wore his best loafers and his feet were no longer swollen.

"You can wear whatever you want here, Peter." It was Silas. He motioned to his t-shirt with a big grin. Peter read it and smiled.

"Sara always wants me to look good. She says, you never know whose watching or who you'll meet up with."

Tara smiled gently and her eyes became even clearer to Peter. "Why don't we walk this way Peter? We have some things to show you."

As they walked forward, the light became brighter still. The colors of the flowers on Peter's left were so vibrant he was awestruck. Lights flickered off each petal and little beings – fairies, fire flies and others he had never see before – danced from flower to flower. The tree trunks blended in with the flowers and purple, green and yellow trees were mixed with dark green leaves. Birds of all species were sitting in them, even birds Peter didn't recognize. It seemed to go on forever.

To his right was the most magnificent desert he had ever seen. The combination of Saguaros and other cacti was incredible. Each was adorned with vibrant flowers, housing birds and providing sustenance and shelter for them. The sage brushes were full of purple flowers and the air smelled of fresh rain.

Ahead of him was a dense forest of pine and aspen trees. He was now able to see deer, cougar and bears, roaming around and all living in harmony. The fields of flowers on the left and beautiful desert on the right melded into the forest in front of him. The road was the only thing that separated any of this vast landscape.

"Look at that! I must have died and gone to Heaven!"

"You have." Silas spoke with joy in his voice. "This is the best place to be. This is Heaven for you. The Heaven you hoped for and anticipated all your life. And there's so much more for you to see and do. We're here to show you around and get you set up for the next phase of your road." He almost giggled with excitement.

"But where is the meadow I saw before?"

"That was just a preview of what's to come." Silas' melodic voice had an immediate calming effect on Peter.

Peter suddenly understood and smiled. "Follow the yellow brick road, huh?" he mused.

"Of course," Yesh answered as Tara began to skip down the road.

Chapter 9

WHEN HE SLIPPED AWAY, SARA could no longer feel him. They had been married for so many years, how could she not feel him anymore? The sun came through the window, illuminating the lines in her face, casting shadows along the far wall. It was supposed to be a beautiful day, but she felt no beauty. What she did feel was pain; pain in her chest, her head, and deep down in her soul. But now it was time to get busy. Time to go through the funeral plans, the mortuary, the service, announcements.

She didn't want to do this, but Brian came along to help finalize the arrangements. Emma had taken Emily home and called Tom, asking him to come home as soon as he could. He had already been on his way when Emma contacted him the day before. The military had given him bereavement leave, acknowledging his need to be with his family.

Brian drove Sara to the funeral home to help her make decisions on what to do next. The mortuary was decorated in dark mahogany. The furniture was big and black. Pictures with dull lights over them hung on the walls. While it was 12:00 noon outside, the lighting inside seemed as if it were night. The decorative lamps on the end tables showed dim light, the hard wood floors were equally dark. The elegant floor rug spoke of expensive Indian design and dark shutters hung heavily on the windows.

This was a business just like the cancer clinic had been which did not go unnoticed by Sara.

David Camden greeted her and Brian in the lobby with a hearty handshake and tempered smile. He was tall, in his mid 50s with graying hair and striking green eyes. His suit was obviously Armani; black and expertly pressed.

"Let me first give you my condolences for your loss. We want to show you the utmost respect here at All Saints Mortuary. Now, shall we sit down in the conference room and go over the necessary arrangements?" He turned and led the way down a dark and dreary hallway.

Sara and Brian took seats side-by-side at the immense table which seated 10. The chairs were huge and nearly swallowed Sara's small frame. They were dark tufted leather and the table cherry wood. Pictures of ducks in reeds nestling on water hung on the wall. Mr. Camden's assistant, Sandra, brought water for everyone. The ringing in Sara's ears intensified to the point she could hardly hear Sandra's voice.

She closed her eyes and asked silently, "Please be quiet so I can hear what's going on here." A moment later, the ringing lessened, but remained in the background.

"Mrs. Hansen," David said, "I have a list of services here we offer our clients. You and your son will want to go over them. We can have the funeral service here or if you prefer you may have the service at a church of your choice. We can also provide services at the cemetery. Whatever you would like."

Brian took the list and began reading. "What do you want, Mom?" he asked as he flipped through the literature. He was exhausted from the last few days but was able to muster up all the compassion he could find.

"You pick Brian," Sara said. "I don't know what to do. Peter was loved by everyone. We should probably do something nice for him and for them."

Sara couldn't look at the paperwork. It was all too much. It was an effort just to breathe. An effort to sit upright in the chair and to walk.

"Mom, look at the costs of things first," Brian said, anxiety rising in his voice. "It's really expensive. Did Dad have any life insurance? I forgot to ask when he was sick."

"Yes. Not a lot but some. I pulled the policy out a few months ago and went over it. They won't pay until we have a death certificate though. Maybe we should ask Emma what she thinks." Sara's voice was heavy with grief.

Mr. Camden interjected, "We can accept a credit card or check for payment. Usually we take one-half down and if there is life insurance we can wait on the balance. Why don't I leave the two of you alone for a while to go over the list of services and make a decision? I'll come back in 15 or 20 minutes." He stood, walking out the door, silently closed the door behind him.

"What are we going to do, Brian? Do we want them to print announcements and order flowers?" Everything was hurting so much; she just wanted this to all go away.

"We don't have to decide right now, Mom. Why don't Emma and I take care of this? We'll let you know what we decide and then you can approve it." Brian ached so much, but he had to push it down so he could be there for Sara. "At least come with me to pick out a casket."

"Your Dad wanted to be cremated and his ashes spread in a meadow. He always loved the Grand Canyon. A long time ago he said that's where he wanted to be when he died. We had gone to the North Rim and found a beautiful spot to camp. I remember exactly where it was."

Sara closed her eyes. She began to visualize the campground and as she did she remembered Peter's description of the meadow from his last hospital stay. The last time they were camping, they had sat on the very edge of the forest, next to an incredible meadow. While she reminisced, taking in the view of the beautiful flowers, it was almost as if she were there.

Suddenly she realized this was the same meadow Peter had talked about. The sounds of the birds and the feeling of the cool breeze on her face were so real. As she thought more about it, the more real it became. She had stepped into the meadow herself. To her right, she saw a shadowy figure of a man standing next to the aspen trees about 100 feet away. Sara strained to look closer and he began to come into view.

"MOM!" Brian yelled. He was tugging on her sleeve, trying to get her attention. "What's going on? I'm talking to you." He was getting irritated and now his patience was nearly gone.

"What? Why are you so mad? Where are we anyway?" Sara looked around the room as if she didn't remember anything about where she was.

"Mom, we're at the funeral home. Where are you?" Brian asked sarcastically. He hadn't slept well in days and it was beginning to show.

"What?" she asked again. She ached to go back to the meadow, to see who was by the trees. "Oh. What are we doing? I think I need something to eat. Why don't we go home? Dad's going to wonder where we are." She wheeled her chair back from the table and stood up to leave.

"Okay Mom. I'll go get you some water and be right back." Brian got up and went to the door. "Don't go anywhere Mom." He had completely forgotten about the water Sandra had brought to them a few minutes earlier.

"Oh, I won't." She sat back down and watched him walk out of the room. "Now, where was I?" she asked herself. "Oh yes, the meadow."

She closed her eyes and took a few slow deep breaths. The meadow began to come into view again. Breathing in the smells of the pine and aspen trees and fresh air, the sounds of the birds, soft at first, began to get louder. The lighting was brighter and the sun shone above her head.

"I'm here," she thought. *"Now where did you go mister?"*

She said referring to the shadowy figure in the tree line. She looked to her right, but the figure was not there. She panned across the meadow but didn't see anyone.

"Where did he go? I saw him just a few minutes ago."

Sadness began to fill her as she realized the man was not there anymore. She thought she recognized him, and was hoping it was Peter, but she just wasn't sure.

"I know you're out there somewhere. I'm going to find you if I have to stay here all day!"

When Brian came back into the room with some water he saw Sara staring out into space. Hastily he had picked out an urn and made arrangements for a service, signed a contract and gave them his credit card. He would run it all by Emma first, and then they would talk with Sara together.

"I've always made more money than anyone, so I'll pay for this," he told the funeral director.

Brian wanted to help but felt helpless at the same time. Taking charge was his way of coping. But now his primary objective was to get Sara home and something to eat. It was distressing having her fading in and out like that. He was not prepared to lose both his parents.

The three of them agreed on a short service, with announcements and a small obituary in the paper. The service was at Sara's church, with Pastor Paul at the pulpit. Many of their friends and extended family came, giving their condolences to Sara, Brian, and Emma. Tom had made it home in time for the service, but his leave was short and he had to return within a week. His tour was ending soon, within the next 9 months, and he didn't want to disrupt his team. He was pulled between staying home and going back. Emma encouraged him to leave, saying she and Emily would be fine, and they had lots to do taking care of Sara now. She was worried for her mom, especially after talking with Brian about the experience with her at the funeral home.

Chapter 10

THE EARLY MORNING LIGHT SHOWN through the little pink and white curtains and onto Sara's kitchen table. She had opened the shutters in the front room when she rose mostly out of habit. It didn't seem right to have the sunlight shut out; but even with the light coming through the windows, everything felt wrong. Everything. Moving felt wrong. Breathing was an effort. Doing anything was exhausting.

Sara set a place for Peter, as she always did. Soon she anticipated hearing him rustling in the next room, clearing his throat as he approached from the hallway. She poured his coffee and placed the wheat toast in the middle of the table and took her place at the other end. Except for the birds beginning to sing outside and the sound of the coffee pot grumbling, silence engulfed her. It was cold outside and inside too. The heater was on but she felt a cold draft beside her.

"Sara?" a pause, then "Sara?"

Sara looked around the room. She heard her name, but not as though it had come from down the hall or from behind her. The sound came from inside her head. It was Peter's voice, clear as the sun shining through the window.

"Sara?"

"Peter? I hear you but I can't see you. Where are you? What's happening?" she was turning around in her chair, looking all around the room.

"One thing at a time, my dear. One thing at a time," Peter said quietly.

"Where are you? You sound like you are in my head. Am I going crazy?" Sara began to wonder what was happening to her. "Are you made up because I miss you so much?" Tears began to roll down her cheeks.

"I am right here with you. Sitting at my place at the table you just set for me." Peter's soothing voice helped to clam the rising fear inside her.

Sara looked at Peter's chair and saw nothing. "I must be losing my mind," she said, shaking her head.

After a moment she heard Peter say, "You are definitely not losing your mind, Sara. Just close your eyes and look again, without opening them."

Reluctantly, Sara did as she heard, closing her eyes. "OK, now what?"

"Just use your imagination. Picture the room, this table, and imagine me sitting in my place."

Sara again, did as she heard. She imagined Peter sitting in his place the last time she saw him there. He was in his robe, trying to drink a cup of coffee, his skin the color of gray, with no hair on his head, eyebrows or eyelashes. As she imagined him he began to take shape in front of her. He was there in her mind, just as she had remembered him.

"Now open your eyes dear," he said quietly.

Slowly Sara opened her eyes and there he was as she knew him before the cancer, before the chemo, before the radiation. His beautiful blond hair was back, neatly cut and wavy. His face was full and his eyes glistened. It was Peter as before, when he was in great health, vibrant and full of life. But something was a little different. He had a glow about him she had never seen before. He radiated beautiful white light which made the room even brighter than it had been.

"Oh God, Peter, is it really you? Can it really be you?" Sara began to cry at the sight of him. Taking a tissue out of her pocket she began to blow her nose.

"Yes, Sara, it's really me." It was almost a whisper, so gentle and so serene.

"Oh God how I've missed you! You look so good!" Sara was in complete shock. "You look better than I've ever seen you. What happened? I thought you were dead! No, wait a minute, I watched you die in the Hospice home, and I saw you in the mortuary!"

Peter waited a moment before speaking. "Well I am what people call 'dead' I guess. I have learned so much. There is a lot more, on the 'other side' so to speak. Things are very different yet the same in many ways."

"Peter, are you saying you're dead but can still talk to me? Can you still see me?"

Sara stopped crying, and started listening very intently. She sat fully back in her chair, squinting, still not believing what was in front of her.

"Yes you could say that."

"I'm not crazy? I always believed but never had any proof! Now here you are."

"Yes. Sara," he said very gently. "And I want to take you with me; to show you some of the wonderful things I have seen. That is, if you want to go. It's not your time to come with me and stay, but you can visit. I can teach you, so when it is your time, you will cross over with no fear at all. Are you interested?"

"Peter I've missed you so much. How could I say no? When do we leave and for how long? Where will we go?"

Sara was beginning to feel energy flowing through her. Energy she never felt before. It was a tingling sensation that stared from her feet and moved rapidly up her legs, into her torso and continued to the top of her head.

Peter looked at Sara with soft loving eyes. He had begun to feel the compassion and love for her he had when they first met. As he focused on this, Sara began to feel it too. She didn't understand where it was coming from but knew it in her heart. Peter truly loved her and wanted her to know all the love and compassion he felt for her.

Sara felt light headed for a moment, and then she seemed to adjust to the energy beginning to flow through her. As Peter focused on the love and compassion, he began sending it her way. She absorbed it slowly at first, but questions began to fill her mind and resistance popped up.

"Peter, how will I get back? Where are we going? Are we going to heaven?"

"Sara, we can go anywhere you want to. I should tell you some details first though." Peter explained. "You won't be taking your body with you on our little trip. You'll have to leave it here. You can sit at the table and we'll just go for a short hop. You see, we are not our physical bodies. We are so much more than that. We are pure energy with the capability of leaving our bodies and going to many different places."

"Does it mean we go to heaven or hell when we leave? How do we make sure we don't go to hell?" Sara asked with growing concern.

"There is no hell, Sara. Hell exists in our minds and which we create in our existence. Many people seem to think we can't have Heaven without having hell. It's not true. Not in God's world that is. Our free will certainly creates hell for some of us and Lord knows many people are already in hell here on earth. That's why if you believe you were 'bad' and are going to hell, you definitely will go to a place when you die you created called hell. But trust me; those who do won't stay there for long. Angels will come to rescue them immediately from such a place. But I'm getting way ahead of myself."

"Alright. I've always trusted you, Peter. I want to go with you. What do I have to do?" Her confidence was growing.

"Just trust you are always safe. Let go your resistance and feel the love in the room. Now take a deep breath and close your eyes."

Sara took one deep breath, and then another. As she closed her eyes she began to feel the energy change again. "I feel so light."

Peter felt the shift in her energy. "Alright. In your mind I want you to imagine you are standing up."

Peter reached for her hand. She took his and she rose out of her body, out of her chair, out of the room and outside with a single gliding thought. It felt as though she was flying yet there was no density to her body. His hand felt strong and secure and she knew she wouldn't fall or be hurt. She never felt lighter.

Crossing from the kitchen to this place took no time at all. Sara felt a whoosh and heard something like a gentle breeze, and they arrived at their destination. Peter had a firm hold of her hand and this helped her feel safe and secure. But it wasn't really Peter who made her feel safe. It was a presence she couldn't identify.

They were standing in the sand at the edge of a river bank, like the portion of the Oak Creek Canyon where they spent the early years of their marriage. The colors were more vibrant than anything she had ever seen before. They blended together but at the same time they had edges to them. It was a beautiful place with tall trees lining the edge on one side and a beach-like setting on the other. There were some high clouds with pale pink and blue highlights.

"Who else is here, Peter?" she asked. "I feel like there are many others here but I can't see them."

"There are others, honey; they just don't want to startle you. Do you remember Sam and Tony? They are here," Peter pointed to his right. "Standing over there."

About 50 feet away from them was a beautiful grassy field dotted with bright orange and yellow wild flowers. Standing in the middle of the field were Sam and Tony, Sara's cousins. They looked as though they were in their mid 30s; handsome and strong, dressed in overalls with blue shirts. Tony smiled and waved. Sara was amazed! How can this be?

"Peter, where are we?" she asked carefully.

"We are on the other side of The Veil, dear."

"The other side of what? What veil? This is the most beautiful place I've ever seen, but it seems too good to be real. And is that really Tony and Sam standing over there? They look too young, not like they did when they died. Oh…they died."

Her voice began to quiver and the fear began to creep into her being.

"Am I dead Peter?"

She felt a whoosh and she was back at the table in the kitchen.

Chapter 11

"MOM, ARE YOU HOME?"

It was Brian. He had just unlocked the door and was walking in when she returned. He had been ringing the doorbell, but she didn't answer. He became concerned and decided to use his key.

"Yes! I'm here," she yelled, shaken.

"Mom I'm right here, you don't have to yell. I've been ringing the door bell for 5 minutes. Where were you?" Brian was somewhat frustrated, again.

"Sitting here at the table, I think. Why are you here?" She was still flustered from the trip.

"Was that an out-of-body experience?" she thought to herself.

Brian came into the kitchen and sat at the table, in his father's place.

"Don't you remember? I came over to help clean out Dad's closet so we can donate his clothes. I'm sorry I'm a little late, but traffic was terrible. Are you ready?" Brian looked at Sara with some concern, eyebrows coming heavily together.

"I guess. Do you want coffee?" She didn't think she could stand yet and it made sense to try to stall him.

"Mom, you know I don't drink coffee. Let's go in the bedroom and get started. I brought some boxes."

Brian surveyed the table and noticed he was sitting in Peter's old space. A cup of coffee was poured and a plate sat ready for a meal. Now he was more concerned about her. He stood up, walking around the table, taking Sara's arm to help her up. She felt a little dizzy for a moment but it passed and with help from Brian she was able to walk to the bedroom. This was another necessary step in the process of saying goodbye to Peter, but it had to be done. Looking at his clothes and putting them in boxes meant he wasn't coming back. He was gone for good. But after her little encounter with Peter, she was beginning to have a different perspective. The thought of having another visit energized her.

She knew someone else could use his clothes. The shelter they supported always needed help. They took families off the street and gave them a new start, providing them with a fully furnished apartment, clothes and a well-stocked kitchen. The adults were helped with finding employment and after three months the family was able to move out and take everything with them. This shelter needed all the donations they could get.

Brian began taking the clothes off the hangers and placing them in the boxes. Sara gathered his socks and underwear and placed them in bags, with tears running down her cheeks. She was going through the motions of cleaning up, taking her love and putting it in a bag.

But what had she just experienced in the kitchen? Maybe she was dreaming; she wanted to be with him so much and had fallen asleep and dreamed he came to her.

"That must be it, it must be."

And what was this silly thing about seeing Sam and Tony again? She hadn't thought of them in years. Tony died so long ago that she didn't even remember when, and Sam had been dead for five or six years of Alzheimer's disease. The memory of seeing them was beginning to fade so it must have been a dream.

"I need a nap," she told Brian after a while. "This is taking longer than I thought and I'm exhausted. Can I just lie down for a while?"

"Sure Mom, I'll finish up. You go lay down on the couch for a while and I'll put everything in my car." Sara shuffled off to the living room to lay down.

Brian was having a hard time with this too. His dad had died and his mom was not doing well. She didn't look good to him; very tired and weak. He thought about calling the doctor for her, just to see if she was alright but then he quickly forgot. The task at hand required too much concentration. The stress was beginning to take its toll on him too.

Dad had only been gone 8 days, but it seemed much longer than that. Time was changing for Brian and he didn't know what to do about it. Everything seemed to slow down. Some days it felt like there was no time constraints and nothing exciting happened. Other days, everything seemed to speed up and the day would be over before it started. He knew he had gone to work and did what was required of him, but he couldn't remember actually sitting down at his desk.

Brian gathered the boxes and began putting them in his Cadillac Escalade. There was plenty of room left over and he considered asking Sara if she wanted to donate anything else. As he walked back into the house, he saw her sleeping peacefully on the couch.

"I'll just be going now, Mom," he gently touched her arm.

"OK, dear. I love you," she responded without opening her eyes.

"Love you too, Mom." He locked the door behind him.

Chapter 12

IT WAS A BRIGHT SATURDAY morning and the air was crisp and cool. Sara and Brian were sitting outside on the patio. Her mood was stoic. All she wanted to do was sleep. She tried to visit with Peter again, but had failed. Emily tried to get her to play, but Sara stared ahead. She made very little eye contact and spoke only a few two or three word sentences. Off in her own world again, was Brian and Emma's summation.

"Watch me Grammy," Emily squealed. "Papa is watching. He says I look like a shiny spinning top!"

Brian watched at Emily. "Yes, you do."

"I wish she would stop this nonsense about Dad. Every day she talks to him like he's here," Brian's emotions were filled with despair.

Losing his dad had taken its toll, much more than Brian had ever imagined. He had been very close to his dad while growing up. Peter always guided his children with a gentle way, never pushing but giving examples of many choices to take when a situation arose. Then he would simply sit back watching them make their decisions based on those examples. If they chose wisely, then he would sit up straight, smile and puff out his chest. If they chose poorly, he would raise his eyebrows and wear an ever-so-slight frown.

"We have to figure out what to do with you now," Brian said not looking at Sara. Immediately he cringed. He knew he had chosen his words poorly and he felt his father's disapproval immediately.

Sara seemed to come back from wherever she was and looked at Brian.

"Do with me?" she asked with sarcasm in her voice, eyebrows raised.

"Papa wants to take her on a vacation," Emily she continued to twirl.

"Do with me?" Sara asked again now with sadness.

"Mom, I'm sorry. I didn't mean it that way. It's just that I worry about you being here by yourself all the time. You don't really drive anymore. You don't have any way to get around...."

"You mean you and Emma have to do for me what your father did. I'm sorry to be such a burden. And, by the way, I'm not alone. Your father comes to visit. We have very nice conversations about you and the decisions you are making. He has a very good perspective on you now." Sara spoke crossly at him for the first time in years. She was not the disciplinarian in the family so this response was very unusual for her.

Angry, Sara stood up to go inside and stumbled on the chair leg. She tried to catch herself by grabbing the table, but missed. She went down hard and everyone could hear the breaking of her hip, the crashing of her head against the concrete.

"Oh my God. Oh my God! Emily, go get your mother now!" Brian screamed as he ran to Sara's side.

Emily darted inside. Sara's face showed her pain, but she had hit her head hard on the concrete and a bump above her eye immediately started to swell. She moaned, but didn't move. Emma came running outside with the phone and dialed 911.

"Emily! Go inside to wait for the fire truck to let them in." Emily ran inside the house and stood watch by the front door. They were there in less than two minutes but it seemed like two hours to Brian.

"I can't believe I did this to you Mom. Please forgive me. I'm so sorry," Brian began to cry.

"What are you talking about?" Emma asked.

"We were talking about what she would do now that Dad is gone. I was mean and made her mad. She got up to go inside and fell."

Brian openly cried for the first time in years. As the firemen arrived, Emily opened the door, leading them to the outside patio. While the paramedics worked on Sara, she lost all consciousness. Emily could see her and Peter standing off to the side.

"It doesn't hurt," Sara spoke quietly. "Why?"

She was standing about 15 feet away, on the other side of the patio with Peter, observing the firemen and the chaos happening before her.

"Because you, who you really are, your spirit, is standing with me. It doesn't hurt now, but when you go back it will. I'm sorry Love, but it's not your time. Brian still has a lot to learn and you are his teacher."

Standing quietly behind them were Yesh, Silas and Tara.

"We brought you over here so you wouldn't feel all the pain and confusion of the fall," Peter explained. "Since our first visit you've been open to the possibility of being where I stand. Now more of your consciousness is with me."

"Brian wants to put me away, Peter. He doesn't want me anymore. He always loved you more than me." She turned to him, looking away from her body and the firemen.

"Why don't I just stay with you now? This is so much better," Sara pleaded, holding on to Peter's arm.

"You can't. I'm sorry. Brian needs to open his heart and his mind. Only with your guidance will he do that. Only with you will he be able to see me," Peter explained. "They are taking you to the hospital now. You have to go back but we'll talk soon. Remember, I am only a breath away."

And with that, Sara returned to her body. The paramedics had given her pain medication so she was asleep, not feeling any discomfort. Her right hip was fractured and she had a concussion. Her recovery would be long and arduous. She was in and out of consciousness the rest of the day, asking for Peter, then Emma and finally Brian.

Finally she slipped into a coma, which was frightening for both Brian and Emma. They kept a vigil by her side taking turns. Emma took the day shift so she could be home with Emily in the evening and Brian stayed at night.

Chapter 13

It took some time, but Sara began to understand the intensity of what was happening. The chills on her right shoulder, the feeling of pressure on her back. It was a light pressure, but she was certain she could feel something or someone touching her. There were soft sounds slowly increasing. Sounds she couldn't explain.

At first she thought it was music, but it was too faint to hear. Maybe it was the sound of someone singing. *No, it's a violin.* Slow, methodical, one note at a time. It was beginning to get louder, but still very faint. Had she heard that sound before?

"No, *it's not a violin, it's a piano,*" she thought. "*I love piano music. How can I be so confused? Where am I?*"

Again, the sound became louder and it was both a violin and a piano. Soothing, soft and comforting. Almost as a lullaby. Hauntingly familiar in its rhythm. It was so beautiful and she immediately began to feel peaceful; her pounding heart began to slow, blood pressure returning to normal. The ringing in her ears was more intense but no longer annoying. The ringing had become background noise.

She was standing in an area with no definition, no corners, and no shapes. There was light, but no objects she could identify, such as a couch or a chair. She couldn't really see anything with form at all. She felt like she was standing in a thick white cloud.

As music came into her consciousness, her vision began to clear as well. What was foggy with little light began to show sharp edges, more defined forms. There appeared to be three people standing nearby. No, maybe more. The more her vision cleared, the more forms of people she could see, but those were standing far away, in the background. The three people who were close to her were becoming clearer.

"Who's there?" Sara asked so quietly anyone near would have to strain to hear her. The music became louder after her question and her vision cleared even more now that she had asked.

"I think I see someone," Sara squinted to see and strained to hear the music, hoping to hear a response from the figures. "I'm not alone, am I?" It was more of a statement than a question.

"No, Dear One, you are not alone."

A soft voice responded in such a kind and gentle manner. While she was not afraid, she felt a quickening in her heart. An outline of a figure standing to her left began to emerge. The voice was within Sara's mind, but also outside of her. It was the voice of an adult male, somewhere in his 50s, she guessed. As he spoke, the music played and an angelic voice began to sing a melody in the background.

"I knew someone was there. Who are you and how many of you are there?" Sara asked a little less timidly than before, still trying to get a bearing on her surroundings.

"There are many of us. We are what some people call The Observers. You have stepped into a place where healing can begin," the voice responded, "Where all things are possible."

"Well, where is that?" she asked, her bravery taking hold. A beautiful crimson couch began to take shape. As she observed it, she took a few steps forward and sat softly, engulfed in its comfort.

"This concept is hard to understand right now but we are here, watching and waiting for people to ask for assistance. It's a place where we observe. When someone asks for help then we respond, in a manner which is appropriate for everyone's highest good."

"Oh. Do you have a name? What can I call you?"

"You may call me Matthew." the voice said.

Matthew began to take shape even more than before, becoming clearer by the moment, materializing before her eyes. He was very tall, at least 6'5", with a slender build, long flowing brown hair and penetrating blue eyes. His clothing was of ancient days and Sara thought he looked as though he walked right out of the Bible.

"Matthew, Matthew, Matthew," Sara paused. "Matthew, my name is Sara."

"Very pleased to meet you Sara." He held out his hand and softly took hers. Smiling, she felt a chill throughout her body as he took a seat beside her. The couch did not move with the weight of his body and Sara could not feel him sit next to her, only the touch of his hand.

"And I'm very pleased to meet you Matthew. Now can you please explain what the heck is happening?"

"I look this way because it makes you feel at ease," Matthew said, reading her thoughts. "You, Sara, are in what some call The Void. It's a place between your earthly consciousness and Heaven. But there are many names for where you are."

"I seem to remember hearing about that, but I don't know really what it is. Can you explain?" Sara's curiosity was beginning to grow, along with a twinge of fear. "I'm not in hell am I?"

"No, my dear, you are not in hell. This is a place where you can create whatever you'd like, learn lessons to help you move along on your journey called life, heal your body, mind and spirit and move forward to understanding what some call All That Is," Matthew answered.

"If I can create anything then can I get my health back? If I want Peter back, can I create that?" Sara began to feel the sadness creeping back into her mind and heart.

"Here you can create things and situations for you, but you cannot interfere with another person's path. What you create here sometimes stays here. It's very complicated." Matthew explained with a soothing voice.

He placed his arm around her. As he did, she felt the familiar tingles she had felt before. By now she had determined she was having another vivid dream. One that must be real, but impossible at the same time.

"But I can hardly see anything. All this fog is keeping me from seeing."

"Just as you wish to see on the earth plane, you can see here. Come, take my hand. I'll show you things that may help you to understand." Matthew stood and stepped to the front of her holding out his hand with a warm and inviting smile.

"But will I come back? Does this mean I'm dead or am I just asleep?" She took his hand, standing with ease. As she did, the couch slowly disappeared.

"There is no death as you understand it to be," he explained. "There are many on the earth plane who talk about spirituality, but they are confused. They have followed ways created by man, not by The Divine. They have written words on paper that have survived for multitudes of years and humanity has blindly followed them. The only truth, real truth, resides in your heart. Get in touch with that and everything will fall into place."

"But how do I do that? I know since Peter died my heart is broken and to feel anything anymore would only bring more pain," Sadness engulfed her when she spoke of Peter's death.

"You are supported in all ways; and you have a very profound connection with Us. The pain and discomfort is your choice. You need not suffer. The Infinite Source dwells within you at all times. Allow this feeling of Source – All That Is – to grow and expand – and you will feel your connection to Spirit. Allowing is the key – allow these gifts, these connections, to take you directly to The Divine, that which you call God.

"The sadness and uncomfortable feelings are merely a stepping stone towards bliss. Allow your own inner Divine connection to strengthen and you will obtain greater peace – peace you have never felt before. Then the sadness, the broken feelings, will fall away and you will become that which you are – connected to the Heart, Mind and Body of The Divine. Receive it now. Every question will be answered and, if not, then you will understand the answer was of no importance anyway. The only thing which does matter is your connection to The Divine."

Matthew took both her hands in his and the feeling of what he was describing, the connectedness, replaced her sadness.

"There are so many different levels of consciousness that it's impossible to comprehend them right now," he continued. "Some groups think the Astral Plane is a place where mischievous spirits reside. Others think The Void is something like a holding tank where if you were a 'bad' person then you go to this place and spend eternity in a sort of nothingness. Others believe there is a Veil that keeps those who are living from seeing those who are dead.

"This place is all of that and none of it at the same time. It depends on your beliefs. This place, to you, is a stepping stone between Heaven and earth. When you are in a sleep state you come here to create scenarios to work out problems in your waking moments. It's really quite impressive if you can figure out how to take back with you what you have learned here.

"It's also a place where we, The Observers, reside. We are the conduits between what some call God, the Universe, Spirit, Spirit Guides, Angels, and energies that have many other names. Those who reside in their heads most of the time need us to connect with That Which Is Bigger Than Us. Or All That Is."

"So if we spend time in our heads, where does That Which Is Bigger Than Us reside?" Sara asked.

"In your heart, Dear One, in your heart." He placed his arm around her again and the familiar tingling returned.

"I feel that! I feel you touching me. I felt that before, when I was afraid and after Peter died. I felt the tingles and somehow it helped me. And I keep hearing this blasted ringing in my ears!" Changing her attitude, she said meekly, "But I'm not really sure what to say about all of this. Am I here for eternity? Is this some sort of school, or what? I guess I'm still confused."

Matthew was gentle and calm while he explained her predicament. "You were uncomfortable in your body anyway and then had the fall. We merely escorted you here so you could heal better with less stress. Brian and Emma think you are in a coma, which technically you are. Or at least your body is. We had a special request to assist you and it's for your highest good for you to be here right now."

"Oh, that must have been Peter. A special request for me would come from him." Sara beamed.

"Well actually, it was a group effort," Matthew said. "You have a lot of people who love you Sara. They are all praying for you. Mostly they pray that you not be in pain and have a full recovery. Do you remember falling?"

"I do remember it a little bit. It seems so far away, so long ago. I can't remember much of anything. It's like it was a dream or some other person's experience. It feels like I was watching a movie. Did I get hurt bad?" She was beginning to get clear in her mind and as her head cleared, so did her vision.

"Yes, actually you broke your hip and took a big bump on the head. But you will heal with time, if you choose to," Matthew explained.

"Oh that 'if I choose to' story, huh? I want to go back and not be in pain. Can I create that?"

"Of course, but it's unlikely. Your belief you must suffer is so imbedded in your mind. It will take some time to change. But we'll help you as much as you will allow us to. First, and the most important thing for you to remember, is you must not let go of hope."

"Lose hope?" she asked. "I did when Peter died. I don't understand why he was taken from me. He visits, but he doesn't stay long and I can't always see him. Are you saying I should hope I'll see him again?"

"Yes, of course. Consider what it is you really want from your life and when you awake you'll be more in touch so to speak, with me, with Peter and the other Observers. Just be patient Sara. Just be patient."

"And the ringing in my ears? My body doesn't hurt, but I still hear the ringing."

"Actually, Sara that is Us. It is the sound we make when we are near, standing right beside you, residing in your heart."

"All right then. I think I'm ready to go back now."

Chapter 14

GETTING HER OUT OF BED was a challenge even with help of the nurses. It had been 6 days since she came out of her coma and she had stopped talking, except to say "Ouch!" or to moan. When the nurses brought her dinner tray, she would only look at it, then stare out the window.

"Ma, you have to eat." Emma picked up the fork, stabbed some vegetables and gave it to Sara. Sara took the fork but her hand shook as she brought the food to her mouth. Some of the vegetables went in, while the rest spilled on her gown.

"Please, Mom, have another bite," Emma pleaded. Sara began the slow process of eating mashed potatoes and mixed vegetables, but left the unidentifiable meat patty on the plate. Even Emma couldn't blame her for not wanting to eat that.

"We've got to get her something she likes," Emma said more to herself than to anyone. "Would you like some vegetable soup?" she asked.

"Alright," Sara said with a smile. "Yes," looking at Emma directly for the first time in days.

"Well, OK then!" Emma nearly yelled. "I'm going right now." She jumped up from her chair and nearly ran out of the room on a mission to find her mom's favorite soup.

"You know she loves you," Peter said. Sara heard his voice but didn't see him right away.

"Where have you been?" she asked. Peter was standing at the side of Sara's bed, smiling at her with pure love in his eyes.

"Right down the hall, Mom," Brian answered.

Sara's gaze went towards the door where Brian stood. He had just arrived when he heard her talking.

She looked in his direction and said a little annoyed, "Not you. I'm talking to Dad."

"Hmm," Brian mumbled as he stepped in the room and took a chair by her bedside. A few moments later Emma arrived with a single serving of vegetable soup, nice and warm, just like her mom always liked. She placed the bowl on Sara's tray and took away the uneaten plate of food in front of her.

Sara looked back to where Peter had been standing, but he was gone. Emma had taken his place with the soup bowl.

"Oh give me that!" Sara said angrily. "I was talking to your Dad and now you've made him leave!"

With a surprised look Emma said, "Okay Mom," and put the spoon next to the bowl.

Brian motioned his head towards the door and stood up. Emma followed him with tears in her eyes as Sara picked up the spoon and began to eat the soup with ease.

"Everything is easy when you are here, Peter."

"You are just learning a different way, dear. Don't be so hard on the kids," he said as he began to materialize in the room again. Peter was becoming stronger and was able to materialize more solid than before and with greater speed.

"This body is old," she said as she ate another spoonful of soup. Emma and Brian peered into the room and observed the one-sided conversation.

"I don't know what to do. First she doesn't talk for days and now she's talking to the window," Brian huffed. "Plus, did you hear how she snapped at me before you came in?"

"Please don't take it personally. She's lost the love of her life and if she wants to talk to him, I suggest we let her," Tears were slowly streaming down her cheeks. "I'm just glad she's talking again, and eating on her own!"

"We'll see how long it lasts," Brian said sharply.

"Please don't try to be so cynical all the time. You never have any hope; never have anything nice to say!" Emma snapped and started walking down the hallway.

Brian came after her, gently grabbing her arm, turning her toward him. "You're right. I'm sorry. Please let's not fight. It won't accomplish anything. We're getting nowhere and it's just so frustrating. Let's you and I take a break, get some dinner for ourselves and try to make this a little better."

Emma hugged him hard and started to sob. She was so tired, so out of breath, out of life. Everything felt bad and with Tom back in Afghanistan, she was left to do everything by herself. She didn't begrudge him, knowing this was the life they had chosen. Most of the time she was able to make the best of it; but now Dad was gone, Mom was in the hospital and everything was so hard.

Brian's guilt at his mom's fall had been more than he could bear. He had taken on this tough exterior to protect himself from his true feelings, those of helplessness and loss of his father and now his mother. He didn't take to change very well, and the events over the last year and a half resulted in constant change. He thought he would adapt better, would have better skills at taking on change, but it turned out it was only in his professional life. His personal life was something completely different.

Chapter 15

"You know I can't release your Mom to go home," Dr. Paramon said, looking at Sara's chart and thumbing through the pages, not wanting to see the pain in Emma's eyes. She was of East India descent, with a small build, long braided black hair and big dark eyes. Her white coat nearly swallowed her. She had been Peter's doctor during one of his many stays in the hospital and she had come to know the family well. They were standing outside the nurse's station across from Sara's room. Brian had gone for coffee.

"Where will she go?" Emma asked.

Her worst fears for her mom were beginning to become a reality. She had promised her mom and dad they would never have to live in a nursing home. It now looked as though she would be breaking her promise.

Dr. Paramon turned her head and looked very intently at Emma. "There are a few good rehab centers I want you to consider. But I have to tell you, I think Sara has the beginning stages of dementia or Alzheimer's."

Out of the corner of her eye, Emma noticed Brian was walking towards them. He was wearing dress jeans and a button down blue shirt. Always the "GQ" of fashion. Emma was dressed in old jeans and a tee shirt with comfortable sandals. When Emma saw him she could swear someone was walking next to him.

"It looks like — maybe — no. It couldn't be," she thought. *"I'm stressed out with all Mom is going through, and she's missing Dad so much. And so do I."*

"Hey Brian, Doc. Paramon has some bad news for us," she said sadly.

"What's that?" Brian's expression turned to fear as he looked from Emma to Dr. Paramon, handing Emma her coffee.

"I'm afraid your Mom may have dementia. I've run some preliminary tests and everything points towards a diagnosis of dementia of some sort. She's going to have to be discharged to a rehab facility and then most likely to a facility which can handle patients who have all stages of dementia."

Dr. Paramon disliked this part of her job, but knew she had to tell them how it was. Trying to give the news otherwise was disrespectful to them and to Sara.

"What tests?" Brian asked. "This talking to herself? It started after Dad died." He began to feel defensive for Sara.

"She's been non-communicative since she got here. She had a concussion but when she came out of it she hasn't been the same and she doesn't have a brain injury from the fall that we can see." Dr. Paramon was trying to be as gentle as possible.

Emma took Brian's hand, feeling her life closing in around her. Mom hadn't recognized her for days now. She was pleasant and would smile when Emma came in the room, but she mostly stared out the window.

"What could be happening?" Emma was trying to make sense of the news. "Where exactly is she? Her eyes are open; she looks at me but says nothing most of the time. I can't seem to get through to her. She did speak yesterday and ate some soup on her own. Isn't she getting better?"

"People diagnosed with dementia have times where they thrive and then slip back into whatever world they seem to reside in. We don't really have any answers. I'm so sorry," Dr. Paramon turned and looked back at her papers.

Brian left the doctor and Emma in the hallway and went into Sara's room, taking a seat in the chair next to her. Sara was lying in her bed watching something outside her window. Her expression was one of peace instead of agitation and pain.

"My parents gave me support to go where ever I wanted. I am so successful with my finances but I'm such a failure at living with my emotions," Brian

thought. "*I don't think I'm even over the loss of Dad, and now this. It's so not fair, so not fair. How am I supposed to deal with the loss of Mom too? So Mom and Emma's God took Dad and now essentially he's taken Mom too. This is just crap! I can't have her live with me and be changing her diapers. I don't know how people do that!*"

Brian sat with his anger while watching Sara. Emma came in to tell him she was leaving to get Emily. "Will you stay with her?" she asked.

"Yes. When you get a minute call me and we'll talk about what to do next," he spoke without looking at her.

"I want to see Pastor Paul. I'm going to call him and let him know Mom's here. I'd like you to take me…if you don't mind." She reached over and kissed Sara on the cheek. "Bye Mom."

Brian nodded, again not taking his eyes off Sara. Emma left him alone with his frustration. Nurses came in and out for the next few hours and Brian began to fall asleep in the chair and to dream.

"This seems to be the longest goodbye ever, doesn't it Brian?" It was Peter, standing next to him as they looked out over a meadow.

"Dad?" Brian asked.

"Yes son. I'm here."

Brian looked to his right and saw Peter standing next to him looking straight ahead. He turned back and saw the meadow. It was like no other he had seen before. The flowers were brighter than any he could remember and the trees were the darkest shade of green that could not be described. The sky was a brilliant blue and dotted with little white clouds.

"This dream is in HD!" Brian acknowledged. By making a joke, he began to feel more comfortable. "And you look 20 years younger. How can that be?" he asked as he turned towards Peter again.

"There is no time here. I can look any way I wish for you to see me, and this is the best way," Peter responded, turning towards Brian. He seemed to glow a soft pink and white color and his smile was comforting to Brian.

"Well if this is being dead, then maybe I should be here."

Peter put his hand on Brian's shoulder. "No, it's not your time. You have to take care of many things before you come here. But Mom's not far off. She does talk to me and we go places only she and I can share right now. It helps her deal with her physical and emotional pain. She gets to know there is more than suffering a broken hip and a broken heart. So be patient with her, son. Show her compassion and just realize this is a part of her road she is traveling."

"Easy for you to say," Brian answered with sadness in his voice. "You don't have to make any hard decisions for her. All my life you showed me things and allowed me to decide what I wanted. Now it's up to Emma and me to make choices for Mom and you're not here to help. What if we make the wrong choice? What if we stick her some place and they hurt her. You hear about these horrible nursing homes that abuse the elderly. I can't put her in one of those, but I can't take care of her and neither can Emma."

Brian began to release all the pain and frustration he had been choking down. For some reason, he felt safe here. He wasn't afraid to show emotion. This place showed him how to feel again.

"Just follow your heart Brian. Quit thinking so negatively and ask for help from God and ask He guide Dr. Paramon. If you still don't believe there is anything after this life, then just remember this dream. Be open to all possibilities. Remember I'm always with you. I am always with you. I am always with you."

Brian woke up startled. He could feel his father's hand on his shoulder and hear his words in his head. Brian sat up straight in the chair and grabbed the first piece of paper and pen he could find, writing down what Peter had said so he wouldn't forget. He thought he was being foolish but needed to do it anyway. Quick, before it fades!

"Be open to all possibilities. Just remember I'm always with you." Brian could hear his father's voice inside his head.

"Wow. OK." Brian looked around the room.

Sara was still watching out the window. Her breathing slowed and she closed her eyes. She was slipping away, but it wasn't her time. For that, she was grateful. She now understood she had more work to be done.

"Still have a little work to do," she said with her eyes shut.

"What Mom?" Brian asked as he stood beside her bed.

"Still have a little work to do."

Chapter 16

St. Johns was a small one-story church, with seating for about 200 and no place for a choir to stand in the back. There were a few buildings outside for Sunday school and related classes. Pastor Paul had an office in the rectory filled with books and ancient bibles.

Brian reluctantly accompanied Emma to see him. The church was Sara's favorite place and she loved Pastor Paul. She went to Sunday service and assisted with the ice cream socials and vacation bible school. Sara's active service to St. John's made her well-known among the parishioners.

"I'm not doing this very well," Emma confessed to Pastor Paul taking a seat at the round table in the middle of his office. She made the appointment to see him after the discussion with Dr. Paramon. Brian drove because she was so distraught, but secretly he wanted to hear what Pastor had to say. Seated next to Emma with Pastor Paul across from them, Brian crossed his arms and frowned.

"Mom's hardly communicating at all anymore. She looks at me and smiles but won't acknowledge anything I say or bring to show her. I'm not sure what to think. I mean, what is the spiritual answer about dementia?" Emma's voice quivered as the emotion of the last several days worked its way up her throat.

Pastor Paul was a favorite among the parishioners. He was of average build, in his early 40s with short brown hair and green eyes. He loved to wear his "street clothes" when he met with those who were seeking guidance. This made him more accessible he thought, more approachable. His goal was to be one of them, setting them at ease when they spoke. Helping them to be comfortable in telling him what they normally kept inside was his goal.

He thought for a moment about Emma's question. While he wanted to reassure her and Brian everything would be alright, he also wanted to tread lightly. He really didn't know her well and she didn't attend church very often. It was Sara who came, and now it didn't look as though she would be back.

After a moment he said, "I believe we are made up of three things; body, mind and spirit. If she is unable to speak, I strongly believe her mind and spirit are intact. She is just isolated within her mind."

"That makes sense to some degree. But she's such a beautiful, loving person. How could God let something like this happen to her? She didn't do anything to deserve what's going on." Emma spoke with extreme sadness, barely looking at him.

"Look guys, our bodies are perishable. Sometimes it's the brain that goes first. Other times it's the lungs, or the heart. When it's the brain, it inevitably changes the person and how they relate to the world. If she had a tumor on her leg, you wouldn't treat her any differently than if she were healthy. You would still visit with her, talk about Emily, talk about what's going on with your husband and yourself. We should not treat her any differently now because she's not communicating. You should treat her like you did before she became ill."

Pastor Paul hoped his words would sink in. He had all too many parishioners who had to deal with this devastating disease. It was like no other illness he had counseled people about. He had parishioners who came to him before the later stages of the disease, who knew they were "slipping." His favorite Bible passage for that circumstance was *Psalms 121:3,* "He who watches over you will not slumber." He would talk to them about who really was in control of the situation and assist them in developing the cognitive and emotional skills to surrendering to what was happening.

"I know my Mom's faith is strong, but where is God in all of this?" Emma asked.

"Watching, guiding, assisting," Pastor Paul answered. "He's sending messengers to watch over you and your family. Sometimes we can't see those messengers, but they are with her and with you too."

"What kind of messengers? Are you talking about the doctors and nurses?" Brian asked with some hesitation.

"Yes, those are a few. But I believe there is more than what we see. In 2 Corinthians 4:18 it says, 'So we fix our eyes not on what is seen, but on what is unseen. For what is seen is temporary, but what is unseen is eternal.' That's why I believe she may be seeing something we can't. Is she talking to people who aren't there?"

"Yes!" Brian said suddenly, leaning forward in his chair and for the first time uncrossing his arms. "She's thinks she's talking to Dad!" Brian's disgust was showing. He had met Pastor Paul before when Sara dragged him to church a few times so he felt comfortable expressing his frustration and anger.

"Well, Brian, in all likelihood she is. There are numerous studies by doctors and theologians that say people can see the dead. Usually it's just after the deceased person has crossed over. Other times it's long after they have died. Many talk about out-of-body experiences when they have died on the operating table, or had a severe trauma to the brain. Some doctors believe it is lack of oxygen to the brain and the patient is hallucinating. But what about the messages and information they come back with? What about the things they see when they are clinically dead?

"There is our perspective and God's perspective," Pastor Paul continued. "Now, I'm going to go out on a limb but I really feel moved to explain this. Do you want to hear it?"

"Yes of course I do," Emma said immediately.

"Go ahead, what can it hurt?" Brian was beginning to lean more towards Pastor Paul; beginning to open up.

"Well, one theory is there is our perspective and God's. God's perspective is above us and ours is below His. Pretty easy concept to grasp, yes?"

Both Emma and Brian nodded.

"OK, so God is up here," he gestured with his left hand, "and we are down here," he gestured with his right hand. "In 'time' we are born, live our life, and die, right?"

"Yes," Emma said. Brian remained quiet, letting all this begin to sink in.

"God doesn't have time. He created time at the same time as day and night were created and therefore time is a dimension of creation, not of God. So we go along our lives in a straight line where we are born, live and die. Theologians believe and teach there is the 'sleep' after we die, when we are buried or cremated, whatever, and then the body is resurrected. Are you following me?"

Both nodded in agreement.

"So, if God has no time, then He sees our lives all at the same time from the beginning to the end. To God, the resurrection comes at the 'time' of our passing. To some of us, we were 'asleep' and woke up in Heaven so to speak, but to God we never slept. We are immediately back with Him, because from His perspective, there was no sleep, because there is no time."

Brian looked at Emma with a total state of confusion in his eyes. Pastor Paul picked up on this immediately.

"Well, let's put it this way then. We, as humans, are the only ones who measure time. Animals have an internal clock so to speak. They know when to eat, sleep, and play on their time. We set clocks that are not internal to move about in this world we created. Your Mom is now more on God's clock than ours. She is half in and half out of this world. When she doesn't communicate and seems to stare into space, she literally is staring into Space; God's Space. She is probably enjoying time, as she would measure it, on the other side. It's not 'time' for her to cross over yet, to wake up, but she's so close she can see both sides now."

"So do you think Dad is experiencing time as we know it?" Emma asked.

"No, not at all. I'm not exactly sure what's going on with him. That knowledge and understanding I don't have. But I do believe he is coming to talk with Sara as a messenger and if you are open, you may have a visit too." Pastor Paul knew he was crossing the line, but it had to be said.

"So what do you think of dreams, when you have a dream about someone who died?" Brian carefully asked. Emma glanced at him but remained quiet.

"God has many ways He talks to us, Brian. I believe He sends messages in many different ways. I believe our loved ones who have died come to us in dreams, in whispers in the wind, by a song on the radio, and by touch."

Brian looked as though he was beginning to soften a little. If that was true, then he'd have to accept the concept of another dimension. That people with dementia were in a different dimension.

"Demented dimensions. How's that for a new topic?" he thought out loud.

"In a sense, yes," Pastor Paul said. "That's what it is, but who are we to call it demented? To them it may be perfectly fine."

"So dementia doesn't exist there either?" Emma asked.

"Again, I don't know exactly what's going on over on the other side of The Veil. And, by the way, it is called The Veil. It's as though Sara can pull aside The Veil and look in to where your Dad is. She's literally seeing beyond The Veil."

"Then all this conversation she is having, all this revelation if you will, is really not an illness?" Emma asked.

"Because it is something we cannot understand completely, then we give it a name and call it an illness. Patients exhibit symptoms, doctors treat it, and some get better – or clearer on this side – with medication. Others do not. Those who are more over there, beyond The Veil, with most of their spirit on that side, do not appear to respond to medication. They just become quiet. They are somewhere where there is no pain or suffering, where I believe there is peace. We see them as suffering, because we cannot communicate with them, and have thus cast a judgment about them.

"Those who are here with dementia and are combative have a different road they are on. It is more difficult for them, and for us, to live with. Medication assists them in calming down and thus enables them to travel to the other side of The Veil. So, in a sense, it is more humane to give them medication that allows them to sleep, than to be in a conflicted or combative state of mind. I know many don't want this for their family, don't want them medicated, but what do you see as better? Conflicted, agitated and angry, or quiet and peaceful? Just ask for guidance and then look to see the signs. They are everywhere. It is possible they must experience this conflict in order to work out things they did while they were here. It's not up to us to judge them, just help them the best we can."

While Pastor Paul desired for this talk to be comforting, for both Emma and Brian, it was a bit confusing. Pastor Paul had explained a lot, but they needed time to absorb it and mostly to come to grips with what was happening. Emma was comforted by the thought her mom was in a peaceful place most of the time, while Brian, not having much background in spirituality, was more confused than comforted. He would think about it and possibly research what Pastor had said, in order to try to get a handle on this. It would take time.....man's time.

Chapter 17

"Yosemite Sam wouldn't do anything like this. There are three big holes you need to work with. There are two that have legal stuff and I don't know what the other one is," Sara was talking in complete sentences for the first time in a long while. "These people are beating me up! They're trying to kill me." She looked at Emma and said, "How about you just take me out of here?"

She faded out again. This was too much for Emma. Sara was talking nonsense where before she was at least having some coherent one or two word conversations. Emma much preferred when she talked to Dad. At least she wasn't as angry.

"This is common with patients who have dementia," Dr. Edward James explained. "She's in her own world. Unfortunately we can't go where she is to help her."

Dr. James was assigned to Sara after Dr. Paramon released her from the hospital. He was in his late 40s and lived and breathed his work. A tall man, with a trim physique, he had allowed patients with dementia to become his passion after losing his mother to the ugly disease at the young age of 58. He graduated from one of the top universities in the US with honors and dove into research and treatment for his patients. There was little room for relationships outside of his work. Many beautiful women had tried to crack his tough exterior, but if they were not in need of treatment, he couldn't even look at them. Being diagnosed with one of the most horrific diseases possible was the worst thing he could imagine for anyone, and he understood the suffering the family of his patients went through.

The new nursing home he recommended was very clean, well staffed and had the appearance of everything her mother needed. Dr. James visited every week, doing his rounds there as well the hospital. But something was not right with the place and Emma couldn't put her finger on it. Maybe it was the overwhelming smell of disinfectant, or the fact no family seemed to be visiting any of the residents whenever Emma was there.

"Those guys over there think I'm stupid," Sara said, sitting in a wheelchair and looking out the big picture window.

"What guys Mom? Who are you talking about?" Emma sat in a chair next to Sara, facing the window too. She couldn't see anyone outside and there were no other residents in the room.

Sara faded out again, staring out the window as she sat quietly. It was too hot to go outside and the monsoon storms were beginning to build in the east.

"This is the hardest part, watching them go like this," Dr. James commented. He was sitting on the couch with Sara's chart, going over her latest vitals and stats. "Your Mom's illness is called dementia with Lewy bodies," he said turning his gaze to Emma. Explaining the deterioration of his patients was one of the hardest parts of his practice.

"What is that exactly?" Emma turned in her chair to face Dr. James.

"There are abnormal deposits of a protein inside her brain. It results in memory problems, poor judgment, confusion and other cognitive symptoms that overlap with dementia. She may have excessive daytime drowsiness, and hallucinations. She may be stiff or shuffle when she begins to walk again, that is if she is able to walk again, or she may lack facial expressions. In about 50 percent of cases, people have a condition called rapid eye movement sleep disorder. This is when most people dream. During normal REM people act out their experiences. In REM sleep disorder, people act out their dreams, sometimes vividly and violently."

"She's never been a violent person. I can't believe she would do that." Emma was becoming more upset.

"You have to remember, she's not the same person she used to be. That's why this is such a devastating disease for both the patient and the family." Dr. James spoke with a mixture of compassion and sadness in his voice. "I wish I had some hope to give you, but I just don't right now. We'll have to keep an eye on her and watch how fast this progresses."

"What is the treatment?"

"Unfortunately there isn't any. We can't treat her for the hallucinations because people who suffer from this form of dementia are extremely sensitive to medication designed specifically for that. She'll be well-cared for here. The staff is terrific and Dr. Sanchez and I are in frequently to check on everyone. I'm sorry I don't have a better outlook for you. It's just the way it is. Dr. Sanchez will be by in a day or two. We keep each other up to date on what's going on so don't worry and you can call me or him at any time." He stood from his place on the couch and walked away, leaving them at the window.

Emma was overwhelmed. She reached over and gently shook her mom's shoulder. "Mom, I have to go before the storms come. Are you going to be alright?" Emma had to get out of there, fast.

"Of course, dear. Your Dad's with me now."

Sara smiled sweetly at Emma and returned to looking out the window. It seemed when she had the delusion of Peter being around, she was at peace. If there was no treatment, she preferred Sara to be hallucinating about Peter. Emma felt better now about leaving her in this new place. It had only been a few days since Sara had been discharged to this home. Brian came the first day but hadn't returned. She knew he would be back, but it would take time.

Emma kissed her on the cheek and turned to leave. Out of the corner of her eye, she caught sight of someone standing by the window. Habit made her turn around to look, but she wasn't fast enough. Whatever she saw had faded, along with her mom's attention. That had been happening more and more.

"*I hope I'm not losing it!*" Emma thought as she walked towards the door. She began to feel a very gentle presence on her left side and a tingling on her right shoulder, like someone had touched her; had put their arm around her shoulder. Emma stopped walking for a moment.

"*There it is again,*" she thought.

She took a deep breath and continued out the door. Whatever the sensation was, it followed her to her car and seemed to leave as she got in. She took a moment to compose herself when she heard a rumbling of thunder behind her. The sound was enough to get her to start the car and move towards the sitter to gather Emily and go home.

"I feel so bad for her Peter," Sara said to Peter as he returned from walking Emma to her car. "I can only imagine." Peter sat in the chair Emma occupied earlier.

"I feel her pain and her sadness, but most of all I feel how out of control she is with this entire situation. It's a learning lesson for her, and without you she'll have difficulty understanding how to just give in to what is."

Peter spoke to her in his gentle way, caressing her hair. "This is one reason you can't come with me now. You are helping her to evolve in ways she never would. I'm going to ask Emily to see if Emma will bring her to visit you. I'll be here at the same time and do a little communicating with our little angel grandchild."

"I don't know who I am without you Peter. How much longer is this going to take?" Sara was beginning to feel despondent. "I'm overcome."

"All I know is when everything is in place, you will be with me. I don't know what all that entails, but we'll do this together. By the way, try to push those voices away from you. You know; the Shadow People."

Peter was referring to the voices that were making Sara confused and angry. When he called them Shadow People, Sara knew exactly what he meant. They had come to her one night in the hospital telling her things that could not possibly be true. Things like Brian was going to steal her jewelry and her money; Emma was really some evil person who wanted to put her away so she could have her house and all her money. Sara knew better but the constant badgering of these voices was sometimes more than she could bear. She began to believe them because they worked on her while she was asleep, when she was most vulnerable.

Peter had come to visit her one night and found them in her room. He quickly made them leave and gave Sara a prayer to say to protect herself.

"They want to poison your mind because they can't see anything but darkness in themselves. If you are poisoned, then your light won't shine as bright. It's hard for them to see when they are around you because of your bright light," he explained.

"What do you mean my bright light?" she asked inquisitively.

"People who are kind and loving at their core emit a beautiful light. They literally light up a room when they walk in. Their consistent smile shines as they walk. You are one of those people." Peter spoke the truth about Sara. Everyone loved her and wanted to be around her.

"Where do the Shadow People come from?" Sara asked.

Peter looked around. All the other residents were in their own rooms or in the great room watching television, while the staff was cooking dinner. It was safe to have this conversation because they were alone.

"They are caught in another dimension between your world and mine. They most likely died in the hospital where you were or in this home and their souls are trapped. Many of them don't even know they are dead. They are confused and angry so they feed on others who are vulnerable. Once they have stolen a piece of your good nature they feel a little better. You could think of it as your glass is full, and they have taken a little of your water to quench their thirst. But when you are ill, you can't fill up your glass as you did before and the more they take, the less you have. Soon, if you aren't careful, you become like them, demented, angry and sad. It's very common with people who have been diagnosed with some form of dementia to have lost their happiness to those souls."

"Is that what I have Peter?" Sara asked in a low voice. "I thought I was really seeing you. How could I be demented?" She began to softly cry.

"Oh honey you don't have to worry about that. You *are* really seeing me. Some people become angrily demented when the Shadow People show up. We have to pray for them; bring them to the Light. People's bodies deteriorate and when they do sometimes the Shadow People come. When people are negative or filled with bad drugs and alcohol, they can't resist them. Not always though. It's a long discussion we really don't have time for, so just remember to say the prayer I gave you. That will keep them away."

Peter didn't want to focus on any negativity. His goal was to keep Sara at peace while waiting for her to fully join him. Focusing on the negative only reinforced it. It was a lesson he had learned long ago. This was almost as hard for him as it was for her, but he understood the reason he was here; to guide her and to help her help the kids. Emma and Brian needed to learn the lessons they had come here for, and it had to be with Peter and Sara's assistance.

"What was that again? I can't remember all if it."

"Let's say it together," Peter gently held her hand. He and Sara began:

"The Light of God surrounds me; the Love of God enfolds me; the Power of God protects me; the Presence of God watches over me; wherever I am, God is."

"It's the Unity Prayer and one of the most powerful prayers ever," Peter reminded her. "Of course The Lord's Prayer is just as powerful but this one adds even more protection when you are in a situation that could be unpleasant." Peter always had a great way of putting things that made Sara feel safe.

"Alright young lady, it's time for dinner!" It was Woody, one of the aids.

Woody was a big burly gentleman who had a heart of gold. The staff loved him because he was strong and could lift any of the residents who may need assistance. Sara's hip was still hurting, but Woody could lift her from her wheelchair and into the dining room chair effortlessly.

"OK, let's go!" Sara said and Woody whisked her away from the window.

Chapter 18

SARA HAD BEEN AWAKENED IN the morning and took her usual position, sitting in her wheelchair in her room after breakfast. She slept hunched over, the lap band keeping her securely in the chair. She awoke, opening her eyes and blinking slowly, trying to focus. As her vision cleared, she could see a large red dog sitting in the doorway.

"Come here fella," she said and leaned over to her left. As she did the dog came up to her, wagging his tail, panting and smiling as dogs do when they see their loved one. Sara stroked his head and he gently licked her arm in long loving strokes.

"What's your name mister?" she smiled. He looked familiar, but she wasn't sure if she knew him. Not getting an answer, she decided it was alright to name him.

"Well then, I'm going to call you Buster."

The dog wagged his tail harder.

"Buster, Buster, Buster," she sang in a melodic voice. "Buster, Buster, Buster."

Buster sat down beside her, leaning half on her leg and half on the chair. Sara looked into Buster's eyes and was finally at peace. He had no collar and felt as though he had just had a bath. He was silky smooth and smelled like baby shampoo. As Sara stroked Buster, her blood pressure began to drop back to normal and her breathing was better than it had been since she was in the hospital.

"So this is what they call pet therapy, huh Buster?" Buster wagged his tail as he sat beside her. He felt very content with her and knew this was where he was supposed to be. Sara worried someone would to come in and take him. She thought he must be someone's dog who was visiting. She didn't remember Brian or Emma talking about this place having any pets.

Nursing home residents often benefited from visits by therapy dogs. The dog didn't have to be social, just his presence was enough. Most of the residents preferred time alone with a dog than visiting with people. They saw doctors, nurses and caregivers almost every day, so just having some alone time with the dog was most likely the best part of their existence. It did take time to get therapy dogs approved for the nursing homes. This home had not applied for one, so where had Buster come from?

She could hear voices down the hall, a conversation between a man and a woman. Maybe they were coming for Buster. She hoped not. This was the nicest thing she could remember, stroking this beautiful dog. She missed her pets. After Peter became ill they had given their dog and cat to Emma and Emily to care for. It had broken her heart, but she had kept it quiet. She knew it was the best thing to do. It was very hard to attend to their needs when she and Peter were in and out of hospitals and doctor offices all the time.

Buster perked his ears up as he turned his head towards the door. He could hear the voices too. He turned back to Sara, gave her one quick lick on the arm and went to the door. As he rounded the corner to his right, Dr. Sanchez came in from the left.

"Well young lady, how are you doing today?" he asked. He was looking at the clip board in his hand with Nurse Angela right behind him.

Dr. Juan Sanchez was a strong man, in his mid 50s and well liked at the home. He had worked hard at his residency at Boswell Hospital. His love for the elderly made it an easy transition to work in the several nursing homes he attended to. Dr. Sanchez had been brought up by his grandmother in Yuma, Arizona. She had instilled a strong sense of values, honesty and hard work in him, which rewarded him with honors in medical school and a place at any hospital of his choosing. Boswell had been a big draw for him. He was an Arizona resident and intended to stay one.

"Whose dog is that?" Sara asked.

"What dog, Sara?" Doc. Sanchez asked as he looked around.

"Buster. Well, at least that's what I call him. He's the red dog that was in here. You couldn't have missed him. He left just as you came in," Sara explained.

"Well, Sara, I didn't see any dog. But maybe I wasn't looking. Funny, I had a dog named Buster when I was a kid. He was the best dog I'd ever had," he reminisced. "Now let's take a look at you, OK?"

"Yes, but I'm feeling much better than the last time I saw you," her voice was clear and her eyes were bright.

"Let's see about that," He pulled out his stethoscope. "Why don't we get your blood pressure?"

Nurse Angela brought out her blood pressure cuff and placed it on Sara's arm while he began to listen to her heart. He inspected her neck, shoulders and felt her pulse in her feet, squeezing gently, looking for any swelling in her lymph nodes. There was none detected and he felt she was doing better than when she first arrived.

"113 over 78 Doctor," Nurse Angela said as she began to write Sara's blood pressure on the chart.

"Well Missy, that's a whole lot better than last time," he smiled at her.

"It's because I was petting Buster. He made me feel really good," Sara was sure of it. "I knew I felt better just by touching him."

"Well we better find this guy and get him to all the residents," he smiled as he left the room.

He was used to his patients hallucinating. To him, this was part of the process of Alzheimer's and dementia in general. There were so many stories his patients would come up, he could write a book just on those alone. He'd call it "Hallucination of the Day" and he was pretty sure it would be a best seller. Actually it was part of why he loved working with the elderly. They had some of the best tales about visitors, traveling, going to the future and back in time. It intrigued him.

"I'm willing to share him. When you find him, please send him back in Okay? I had a dog like him when I was a little girl. My sister called him Red of all things, but I like the name Buster better."

Sara was reminiscing again; the only problem was she never had a sister. Doc. Sanchez and Nurse Angela didn't know the details of her siblings so they just nodded and smiled. She was beginning to move from one universe to another, and trying to keep them straight had become a challenge. When she was "over there" things were different. She had other family and friends. It was confusing, very difficult to keep things in perspective.

"Sometimes we switch between over there and back here a little too fast." It was Peter. He was standing next to her and he placed his hand on her shoulder.

"What do you mean" Sara asked.

"Well, you were sleeping and as you were sleeping, your body remains here, while your spirit travels. Most of the time, we come back to our bodies before we wake up; other times we wake up half here and half over there. What happened this time is you brought Buster's energy with you back to this 'time.' He didn't actually come here with his body, but the essence of who he is came. Because you were half here and half there and Buster was over there, when you returned or woke up, you were able to feel him as though he was really here."

"Is that why Doc. Sanchez couldn't see him?" She was beginning to understand the difference between two universes and traveling between them.

"Yes. Doc. Sanchez hasn't experienced over there like you have. He has dreams, some of which appear to be very real to him, but he's not interested in exploring them further. He thinks they are just dreams. To him, they are meaningless. He has been taught they are of no significance, just like most people. It's hard to believe in something you can't see when you have been told something else all your life by people you trust."

"So, when you are here with me is it a dream for you?" Sara asked

"No because I no longer have a body. This makes my ability to move from here to there instantaneous. I am in Spirit now, so I can travel anywhere I want to go; this place with you and other places you can't even imagine. It's so beautiful in some and so amazing in others. You can stand on the moon or stand on another planet. It is limitless and quite unexplainable." Peter explained.

"Why can't I just go with you now? I hate this body. I hate feeling this now. I can't do anything anymore. I can't even walk!" Sara was beginning to get agitated, and loud.

"Just be patient, Sara. Just be patient."

The nurses heard Sara and began to come down the hall to her room. They rounded the corner and as they entered her room, Sara stopped talking.

"Sara, what's up honey?" Nurse Angela asked. Tracie, the nurse's aide on staff, was with Angela and right behind her as she came into the room.

"I want out! I just want out!" Sara was inconsolable. "Please let me out!"

"Sara," Angela said softly. "You can come out. Let's go out on the patio. It's a beautiful day and the patio is so pretty. Tracie, will you bring Sara outside?"

"I'd be happy to. Come with me Sara," Tracie said.

She was a beautiful young black woman; tall with a slim body. She could lift twice her weight and she loved the residents. Her parents wanted her to be a doctor, her older brother thought she should be a professional singer because of her lovely voice, but she wanted to be of service to those less fortunate.

As Tracie wheeled Sara out of her room and down the hall, Sara saw Buster leading the way. Immediately she calmed and started to smile.

"Buster, Buster, Buster," she began to say and repeat as she was wheeled outside. Buster led the way and once outside sat beside her, panting and smiling, licking her arm.

"Thanks Buster."

Chapter 19

Emma had listened to music all her life and lived it, just like her mom. The lyrics of sad songs were prevalent for her. When she had been despondent the lyrics fit her mood. Every now and then when she was feeling blue, she would play one about surrendering and sometimes cry. But now they had a new meaning; one of wanting to release her mother's relentless nightmare of existing in a body which no longer served her. One of wanting to release her mother's mind and let her go.

"I cannot understand why she hangs on. I cannot comprehend it at all!"

Emma had been frustrated for a long time, but it was now coming to the point of anger. She was sitting at her kitchen table after putting Emily to bed, looking at the screen on her computer.

"I understand what Pastor Paul said. I get it. So when is it time to let it go? If I could, you know I would let you go Mom."

Emma had researched dementia on the internet, hoping to find something that would help her mom. She remembered her grandmother going through this but it was so long ago and she was a young teenager, not interested in what was happening to older people. She had regrets about it now. They had so much wisdom and she had missed it because she was young and self-centered.

What Emma had learned was every day was a gift, and love was to be given unconditionally. She had appreciated what she had in her life but with Mom having these problems, with just losing her father; it was all so awakening, such a revelation of just how short life was. Now she realized her responsibility to Emily, to Tom, to Brian. She had to be the person who appreciated life and speak her love for all of them. If she wanted to see that in others, she had to be the example. And the most difficult part was if they did not respond in kind, she would have to overlook it.

"Wow. I always thought if I gave something to someone, or gave of my time, I was supposed to get something in return. That's the way it works, right? But it's not right after all. I think I get it now. I should give and not expect anything in return. What I get in return is the joy on the person's face or the change they may experience.

"I've watched people give a gift to Emily and she just squeals with happiness, she doesn't give them a present in return, she gives them her delight. So, this is how it should be. I also need to remember, once a gift has been given, then to completely give it, I should never mention it again. I understand this is the way to completely give."

Emma had a friend who was very generous. She always did things for others, but she had to have recognition in return. "Did they like the cheesecake I made? Did you like the flowers I brought for you?" Even though the receiver would say thank you, she needed additional pat on the back in order for her to feel better about the gift; to feel better about herself.

Emma didn't want to judge, but she saw the frailty in the need for recognition. The gift no longer was unconditional; it was conditioned upon her friend receiving recognition. Although she didn't begrudge her friend, and realized she was giving from her heart, Emma understood this was not the way she felt it should be.

"We were taught God wanted us to say thank you for our gifts. We were required to say thank you to make God happy." Emma was beginning to realize to be in appreciation of the gifts God gave us was a very strong testament to acknowledging His presence. He didn't expect us to say thank you or needed to have recognition as her friend did. He was happy no matter what, because He exists in a state of continual bliss. That is all He wants for us. We don't make him sad or unhappy, those are human emotions, and to attribute human emotions to God was to make him "feel" anger, frustration, condemnation, revenge. All this was just not possible.

Staying in a mindset of gratitude made her feel better and more at peace. It just felt right to say thank you every morning and to look around at all the greatness there was in the world. Of course there was sadness surrounding her, even outside of what was happening with Mom. There was tension in the world, the economy had taken a dump a few years ago and was still struggling to regain some composure. But what she observed was the good that had come from the problems; people were motivated to make changes and change did not come from complacency.

So, in finding the frailty in her friend's need for recognition, Emma realized she was judging her, and in doing, she became like her. How confusing it was; but at the same time it made sense. WWJD? She loved the phrase; what would Jesus do. Now she was going to step it up a notch and say WWGD? What would God do? God would continue on about his business, not judging her friend at all, just loving her and delighting in the excitement of receiving His gifts. But wasn't that what she was taught about Jesus too?

"If I am to find peace, then perhaps my new saying should be WWGD. I think I'm starting to get this stuff!" she said to herself. "But getting it and doing it are two different things. I need to catch myself every time, or at least almost every time, I fall back into the old ways."

"It's called having a human moment," Peter whispered in her ear.

Emma quickly looked around."Where did that come from?" she asked quietly.

"Dad?" she asked, hearing no response.

She waited a few moments and then asked again, "Dad?"

Silence.

"I must be losing my mind. No, wait a minute. I'm catching myself slipping back into the 'human moment.' Thanks Dad!"

Chapter 20

"Papa! Is that you?" Emily squealed.

Emily was playing in her room after dinner dressed in her pink and white pajamas; the ones with the feet. She began running around in huge circles at the sight of Peter. He was sitting on the end of her bed, wearing his jeans, t-shirt and a big smile.

"Yes, little one, but shhhhh…. You don't want Momma to hear you. Now, I want to talk to you about something."

"Watch me, Papa!" Emily began spinning around the way she had the day Sara fell. "I look like a spinning top, right?"

"Yes, yes you do. Now please sit down on the bed with me and listen. I have a Very Important Mission for you to do. Are you ready?"

With the words Very Important Mission being said, Emily snapped to attention and sat directly on the bed next to Peter. Very Important Mission was the game they played when Emily would visit Peter and Sara. It required following strict instructions on each of their parts. Emily would instruct Peter to find a pair of socks and a hat; then bring them to the middle of the living room. Peter would tell Emily she had to find a piece of paper and a pencil and write her name on it. Each Very Important Mission would always end with Emily learning something.

"Okay Papa. I'm ready," she said with a huge grin as she plopped herself on the bed.

"Well, first this has to be a secret. You can't tell anyone you are playing the Very Important Mission game with me."

"Okay!" Emily loved secrets. She had learned to keep them when her daddy began insisting she didn't have imaginary friends.

"Okay. Now, you have to follow the Very Important Mission instructions just as I give them to you. First I want you to go find Momma and tell her you have to see Grammy tomorrow. It's important you convince her you absolutely positively have to see Grammy tomorrow, Okay?"

"Okay!" Emily jumped off the bed, but Peter motioned for her to sit.

"Wait, wait. There's more," he whispered, trying to temper her enthusiasm just a bit.

"Really?" Emily's eyes got really big.

"Yes. When you get your Momma to bring you tomorrow to see Grammy I'm going to be there too."

"Oh boy!" she squealed. Emma was used to hearing Emily talk to herself, so any noise coming from her room was not surprising at all.

"Yes, and you and I are going to talk to your Momma together. I'm going to say things to you for you to tell your Momma so she will know I'm right there with you. And I want Uncle Brian there too. Sound good to you?"

"Of course. I want Momma to see you too," Emily had just about given up on anyone ever believing her.

"Well, she may not be able to see me tomorrow, but I sure hope she knows I'm there."

"Why don't we do it now? I can go get her." Emily was getting excited about the possibility of Peter being seen by others.

"She's not ready to see me just yet, little one. Let's wait until tomorrow when Grammy is there too because Grammy sees me. Now go on your Very Important Mission." As he patted her gently on the back, she could feel tingling in her shoulders.

"Okay, but you better wait here to see what she says. Sometimes she says no," Emily complained.

"Yes. I'll wait. Go ask."

Emily left her room and danced in little pirouettes as she came down the hallway and into the living room. Emma was sitting on the couch staring blankly at the television. It had become impossible to concentrate on anything and reading was out of the question. She and Emily had a light dinner an hour ago, the dishes were cleaned and put away and she had talked to Tom for a very short time on the internet. The stress of her mother's illness and Tom being in Afghanistan was beginning to show on her face. He had been in town only for a week to assist with getting Sara situated and then had to leave again. Seeing Emily dance into the room made her smile.

"Momma, I have a Very Important Mission." The sound of those words took Emma by surprise. She hadn't heard her play the game since before Peter had died.

"A Very Important Mission? What could that be Em?"

"I want to see Grammy tomorrow," Emily said as she continued to pirouette around the room. "I want to see Grammy tomorrow. I want to see Grammy tomorrow."

"Okay, stop and sit down next to me," Emily was making her dizzy.

"Okay Momma." Emily finished her last circle and sat on the couch. She was dizzy herself.

"What makes you ask about Grammy?"

"It's a Very Important Mission. I have to see her tomorrow."

Emily remembered the secret part but thought she was safe saying Very Important Mission because she didn't say it was Papa she was playing with.

"I don't know, Em. I'm not sure what time I'm going, but let me think about it, Okay?" Emma was exhausted and had been considering not going to visit tomorrow.

"And, I want Uncle Brian to come too. You have to ask him, you have to! Don't think too long. If you do you'll talk yourself right out of it." Emily knew if she couldn't get an answer right away, the answer would eventually be "no."

Emma gazed at Emily intently. Those were Peter's words coming back to her. He would coach her when she had a difficult decision to make and say that very thing. Emma was very adept at over-analyzing things to the point of inaction. How could she resist when she heard that?

"Alright, I won't think about it anymore. I'll take you tomorrow." She caved in to the request quickly.

"Yes, Yes, Yes!"

"Now get ready for bed silly girl!" Emma scooted her off the couch.

"Don't forget to call Uncle Brian. He has to be there too!" Emily said.

Emily ran squealing down the hallway to brush her teeth and hair. When she got back to her room Papa was gone.

"It's okay; I know he knows I did it. Besides he's on a Very Important Mission too."

Chapter 21

"WHEN I THINK OF HEAVEN I think of dying. So do I want to see Heaven? Yes. Because I don't really believe I'm dying the way we learned to think of death," Sara remembered her conversation with Matthew. "We don't die, we move on; we just step out of our car so to speak. Someone has died. So what? The rest of us are left to ourselves, which can be very distressing at times. So how do we let people know how moving out of this body is not the worst thing in the world?

"How do we transform our beliefs to allow us to find the Truth? And what is Truth? Is this just the ramblings of a demented old woman who no longer wants to communicate with those around her? I don't know. Maybe. Maybe I'm speaking the one and only Truth.

"So I've heard prayer and meditation; sitting quietly, removing ourselves from the chaos that ensues when we observe the news, observing our partner's behavior, observing our neighbor's behavior, is one way of getting to the Truth. But whose truth? Christian truth? Jewish truth? Muslim truth? How are we supposed to know which Truth is THE Truth? Isn't this question what causes wars? Don't we fight over whose 'truth' is right and whose 'truth' everyone should believe in?

"I think whatever gets you 'there' is what is the Truth. And 'there' is where love resides. All this fuss and separation only gets us away from the real Heaven. Peaceful conflict resolution is the only way, but I see people spouting this as they talk against others who do not believe their 'truth.' So who is confused here? Who is really demented? How can you say all you want is peaceful conflict resolution when you condemn others for their beliefs – especially if they attack your 'truth' with their 'truth'? Where is the peaceful resolution in that?

"The bottom line is we belong to the Father. We belong together. We are a part of the Divine who resides in our hearts. So if you really want peaceful conflict resolution, you must not condemn others when they attack you or your 'truth'. You absolutely must forgive, as God forgives. You must love as God loves, or at least as close as you can get to God's love and forgiveness. This is the only way we will survive; we must live as One World, instead of this damn separation!

"Can't you hear it? Can't you hear the beautiful music from all nations? Can't you see the incredible inventions from all nations that have been given the chance to have education, the opportunity to express themselves? Can't you see we must acknowledge all creation, all inventions, no matter where they come from? Can't you see the beautiful artwork that expresses the inner workings of the Divine?"

Sara sat in her wheelchair, contemplating these things. She was in the living room and she could hear the news on the television in the great room. She gazed out the big picture window at the birds hovering around the feeders, the roses blooming, the purple iris standing tall with their blooms ready to explode into nature's wonder. This place had a spectacular array of flowers and color. The caretakers were very meticulous about the gardens. They believed it brought peace and tranquility to their residents and the families.

She had withdrawn because speaking required too much energy. It was hard enough just to get in and out of bed. Everything hurt. The discs in her back were beginning to fuse, the swelling in her feet made then unrecognizable. The pain was relentless. Morphine had become the drug of choice. It didn't really remove the pain, just made it more bearable, but it also messed with her head.

"Are these the ramblings of a woman on drugs? Maybe so. Maybe these thoughts are the ramblings of a woman who is no longer demented, but wishes to be left alone, wishes to be out of this painful body, wishes to be with my beloved, wishes to finally see God and all that was promised to me from the church, all that was promised to me by Pastor Paul when he would stand at the pulpit and talk of God. I was promised some things. I believed because of the promises. I think it's time I was delivered those promises."

"Sara, honey, let's go get some lunch, Okay?" it was Nurse Angela, again.

"Why don't you get some lunch and leave me here?" Sara thought as she looked up at Angela. *"She's just doing her job, I know, but if I eat it only keeps this old painful body going. I don't want to eat. It is so humiliating having someone feed me. Like a baby. I can't even say no anymore. And most of all I don't want Angela to feel bad."*

She took a deep breath and grinned her little grin. "Okay, I guess. I'll go."

Angela stepped behind Sara's wheelchair, humming sweetly as she wheeled Sara into the dining room. The unbearable move from the wheelchair to the dining room chair had stopped a few days ago when the only sound Sara made was "OWWWW!! God damn it!" It became clear to Angela, and the other caretakers, it was time to stop this portion of the routine of normalcy and allow Sara to stay where she was. Lunch would be over soon and she would be dismissed to her room to "rest."

Resting consisted of getting her out of her prison wheelchair, onto the bed, a change of diapers (another humiliating experience) and turning on the television. The home had a movie channel consisting of old westerns, Fred Astaire and Gene Kelly movies. They put this on for her at the request of Brian and Emma. "We know she always watched those with Dad," was Emma's request.

Minutes staring at the TV turned into hours which turned into a diaper change, getting back into the chair and heading out for another meal which only prolonged her existence. Pain and suffering. She had not been promised this. Of that she was certain.

"No one promised getting old was easy. That I remember. My mother used to say getting old was torturous. It must be a mistake. She was strong woman, but I remember watching her sit in her damn wheelchair not saying anything, just staring. I think I know why she did that. I get it now. It was an escape from this life. I like that. Peter, I want to escape again. Please come and take me away."

Peter appeared after dinner. "You've been busy," he said.

"Busy? Doing what?" she asked somewhat sarcastically.

"Contemplating the Universe."

"Oh, yea. And was I right about any of it?"

"You did get a lot right. Especially about the peaceful conflict resolution and the separation humans have created. It's all about getting back to where we came from. Getting back to the bosom of God, so to speak. We are all homeward bound. Even me. I'm on a road to home, doing some work while I'm waiting for you."

"What kind of work are you doing, Peter?" Sara asked, her demeanor having calmed to the sweetness of who she really was. Peter's presence always did this for her.

"I've been working on getting Emily to do what she does best, gathering the troops. She's getting everyone together and is on a Very Important Mission," Peter smiled.

"Oh Yes! She loves that!"

"They will be visiting soon. No worries. I've got it all planned out, ha ha," Peter mused.

Sara giggled at this. She knew any plans were made to be changed especially when it came to the kids. Brian could easily get sidetracked, while Emma was always late because she had timing issues. Emily just went along with the flow. Nothing bothered that little one. It was good to know they were coming whether they were on time or not.

"Anything I need to do to prepare?" she asked.

"You're already there. Again, no worries. Good night my love." And Peter faded away.

"Good night dearest."

Chapter 22

"The Light of God surrounds me. The Love of God enfolds me. The Power of God protects me. The Presence of God watches over me. Wherever I am, God is." Sara began to chant the prayer. It was late, after 11:00, and all the residents were asleep.

The Shadow People were lurking in the hallway. They couldn't come in the room while she was saying the prayer, and soon they lost interest in her. Some of them had come to the nursing home, attracted to Sara's light, hoping to find some for themselves. There were a total of eight Shadow People. Bob and David and one of the women, Jane, were a little more aware of the light than the others. They appeared as shadows darting in and out of the peripheral vision of people working there.

The new people at this nursing home attracted the attention of Bob, David and Jane. They had a dim light but there was a light nonetheless. The older man in the room down the hall was one of these people. Hank was his name, but he already had Shadow People attached to him. They glared at the newcomers from his door way. There was no way they were going down the hall with those guys already in there.

"Why won't she stop saying that? I wanted to talk to her." Jane complained of Sara.

Jane had been a miserable person while she was alive. Constantly complaining and blaming everyone for all her ailments. When her family would call and ask how she was, all she could do was to talk about the new pain her in her body and how someone else in the family had disappointed her. She was in her late 70s when she died. Unfortunately her family was relieved and they felt guilty about it at the same time. But at least the complaining had stopped.

"If she's going to keep doing that I'm leaving!" shouted Bob.

He was worse than Jane. He was continually angry and resentful while alive. His favorite past time was drinking cases of beer and beating his wife and children. Humiliation was his power and when he wasn't physically abusing his family, he verbally knocked them down. He was a heavy smoker and died of a heart attack in the ER at the age of 58. No one attended his funeral except his immediate family. Everyone who knew him was relieved he was gone. The heart attack had put them out of their misery.

"I'm going back to the hospital. At least there are more people there. Everyone here is taken!" David said with his usual resentment.

David had been such a slob during his lifetime. He had no ambition, lived with his parents until they died and then lived in the same home until his death. The house was in shambles. He never cleaned anything and garbage was piled high. He died of boredom and complacency. It took several days after his death before anyone even knew he was missing. If it hadn't been for the newspapers and mail piling up outside, it would have been much longer. The city eventually condemned the house.

Sara chanted the prayer until she fell asleep and Peter came to her in her dreams. "Don't forget, I've got Emily coming tomorrow with her mom. I'm going to work on Brian tonight to see if we can get him to come too."

"Yes, I remember. It will be a family reunion. Thank you for the prayer, Peter. The Shadow People were waiting for me outside of my room. I could see them peaking in and out from around the corner. I hope they aren't here anymore."

"Oh they are gone. Don't worry about that. If you ever start to feel insecure, or unsure of anything, just chant the prayer. It works every time."

Sara woke early the next morning in anticipation of the visit from Emily, and of course Emma and Brian. Emily always had so much energy and made her feel better. The Shadow People had moved into some of the resident's rooms who were sleeping. They were talking quietly to them, trying to see if they could get them to share their light. Bea, who was a long-time resident, spoke up very loudly.

"You need to get out of here. I know who you are!" she shouted.

The workers just ignored Bea's outbursts. They were preparing breakfast and decided they would deal with her when it came time to bring her to the table.

"Boy, you don't have to be rude!" It was Bob. It was the last insult he was going to take today. "I'm going somewhere else. Besides, I want a beer. This is a total waste of time. You can't get through to this woman. And every time I try to slap her to get her attention she blocks me. What a pain in the ass. Reminds me of my ex-wife."

"Well you're never going to get a beer in this place. I don't see any alcohol anywhere. What a drag. I think I'll go with you." David had enough of Jane too. She was such a putz, always holding back, hardly ever coming forward to talk to these people. Since the two were in agreement, they quickly disappeared. Jane decided to stay. That Bea woman reminded her of herself.

"You have COPD too! I coughed for years and never smoked. It was my husband and the kids who always smoked around me. That's why I was so sick. They never went outside. The house smelled all the time. No one would listen to me. It's as if I wasn't even there. I had to do all the cooking and cleaning and they would just mess it up again." Jane was on a roll, and Bea was right behind her.

"You think you've got it bad, your family didn't put you here!" Bea said. "They hate me here; always telling me to do this and don't do that. They think I don't have a brain! This is the worst place ever. They threw me out of my own home, just because I wanted to go for a walk. As if I can't go for a walk by myself anymore. And that little one, the one that comes here to visit that Sara woman; she's a little pain in the butt. She dances around so much it makes my dizzy. I here she's coming again today. You better watch out. She'll be able to see you."

"Well, if she can see me then I'll just give her a piece of my bind, I mean my mind. Oh well, I better not give her too much or I won't have any mind left."

The workers came to get Bea ready for breakfast so Jane went down the hall looking for Hank. His Shadow People had a grasp on him and wouldn't let go. Hank was already at the table waiting for breakfast, but they had surrounded him on either side and behind, again glaring at Jane.

"You better stay away. He's ours!" the one standing beside him to his left spoke sharply.

"Who's yours?" Hank asked.

"You are, you nut case," another said.

"I don't want him anyway. Men are such problems. You can have him," Jane scoffed.

"Sara, who has you? If nobody does, can I have you?" Hank asked.

"*I'm a married woman!*" she scolded.

Softly she began to say the protection prayer. The workers thought she was talking to herself again as they placed her eggs and toast in front of her.

"Do you want some fruit Sara?" It was Dana. She was one of the aids who spoke fluent English. The house was run by a Romanian woman who kept a tight ship. Very clean and orderly was her way.

"I was always the one to do that," Sara said. What she meant to say was "yes" but it didn't come out.

"*Why can't I just say what's on my mind?*" she thought to herself. "*Where did that come from?*"

This confused thinking had taken her mind away; her ability to communicate was something she had always been proud of. Now she was beginning to think pride was a deadly sin.

Dana put the bowl of fruit down in front of Sara anyway. "You have some if you want it," she said sweetly and continued to serve Bea and Hank.

Chapter 23

"Your granddaughter is going to be here any minute. You've got to get ready," Dana gently nudged Sara's shoulder.

Sara moved slowly but with purpose. She had suffered through another agonizing lunch and was lying in her bed. Had she heard Dana say something about Emily? It was possible, but she wasn't quite sure what it was she had said. Maybe Emily was coming for a visit. Maybe she would take her away from here. The sooner she was dressed and on the patio, the better.

It was getting harder and harder to get to and from the wheelchair. Dana and Angela worked together, tugging and pulling gently on her arms and torso. They would get her in an upright position on the bed, swing her around by grabbing her legs and pulling them to the edge of the bed and let her rest.

"Oh, god damn it!" was Sara's response.

Every day, every night, they never stopped moving her. She just wanted to lie in bed; she just wanted to sleep, perhaps forever. Finally she was in her chair. Dana wheeled Sara outside and onto the patio. It was a beautiful afternoon, just the perfect temperature, with a little breeze. Sara relaxed as soon as she was outside.

The doorbell rang and Emily ran through the door as soon as Dana opened it.

"Grammy!" she squealed as she ran through the living room and out the back patio door. She nearly jumped in Sara's lap, until Emma pulled her back.

"Be careful!" Emma scolded. "You might hurt her."

Emily didn't mind. She knew Sara was just fine. She heard the doorbell again and in a few moments saw Brian.

"Uncle Brian!" Emily squealed and jumped into his waiting arms.

"Man, you are a breath of fresh air, as they say." He hugged her and spun her around in a circle. "Oh! You're getting too big to do that!"

"I am growing, aren't I?" Emily whispered in his ear.

He carried her outside and put her down as soon as he could. Brian bent down to give Sara a kiss on the cheek, and leaned over to kiss Emma as well. He sat down on the bench next to Emma and said, "Okay, what's up Emily? Why did you want us here so much?"

"Papa asked us to be here." As she said this, Peter began to materialize next to her. Sara immediately responded to the sight of him.

"Oh, Peter. What is going on? I haven't seen you in so long." Sara said with sadness in her voice.

"Tell your mommy and Brian Papa said to be open to all possibilities."

"Papa says to be open to all possibilities," Emily repeated.

She stood very straight, very tall, and spoke with purpose. She seemed to mature before their very eyes.

"Emily…" Emma's voice faded. As she looked at Emily, she could see a faded light next to her. She looked towards the light but it seemed to fade even more. When she looked back at Emily it became clearer.

"Papa says to wait a minute and you can see him better."

"Brian, do you see what I'm seeing?" Emma asked as she turned towards where Brian was sitting.

"What the hell are you talking about?" Brian was beginning to get angry at this exchange. He leaned forward in his chair, tilting his head and looking at Emma with a "what the hell is the matter with this child" expression.

"Uncle Brian, Papa asked you to be open to all possibilities. He said he heard you the other day when you asked what you were supposed to do. He wants you to be open….okay, Papa, he wants you to be aware. What does aware mean Papa?" Emily paused for a moment, looking in Peter's direction.

"Aware means to be sensitive; to see what is going on around you." Peter explained.

"Oh yeah," she said as she turned towards Brian. "Uncle Brian, he wants you to see what's going on around you."

Brian had a perplexed look on his face. His eyebrows narrowed but his hard demeanor began to fade as he sat back in his chair. "How do you know what I was doing the other day Emily?"

"I don't know Uncle Brian, Papa knows."

"Oh, sure, Papa," Brian said somewhat sarcastically. "Papa knows."

He sat even further back in his chair. But there was something familiar about those words, and he began to remember his dream where Peter had said to be open to all possibilities.

But Emma ignored all of this. As long as she looked at Emily, the light was becoming brighter and the shape of a person was beginning to emerge. Every time she looked directly at the light, it went away.

"I'm open and aware, Emily. What else does Papa have to say?" Emma asked.

"What else, Papa?" Emily asked.

"Tell Uncle Brian he doesn't have to be tough anymore. That demented dimensions aren't really demented at all. Ask him to remember talking to Pastor Paul." Peter was trying to get to Brian in a way that he would understand.

"Uncle Brian, Papa says demented dimensions aren't real."

"Where did you hear that?" Brian gasped. He suddenly remembered his conversation with Pastor Paul a while back.

"Papa said it." Emily was beginning to tire of this conversation. "He says they aren't really demented at all and you should listen to Pastor Paul. Papa, can I go now? I want to play."

"You go play, I'll talk to Papa," Sara said. She was witnessing the entire exchange, feeling Emily's need to play. "But stay close by."

"Oh I will. I don't want to go inside where those other people are. That Jane lady is mean and I don't like the others either." Emily had been watching the Shadow People in the window watching her. "Besides, I want to play with Buster!"

"Just stay out here on the patio," Emma directed. She couldn't see the Shadow People, but she was aware of how much trouble a little one like her could get into.

"Mom, I think I see Dad standing over by the pillar. Is that where he is?" Emma asked quietly.

"Yes he is. Now Brian, before you get up disgusted with me again, remember, just because you can't see something doesn't mean it's not there. Remember, you can't see the wind but you can see the effects. Why not just take a moment and consider the possibility." Sara's clarity was amazing. It was the most lucid conversation any of them had had with Sara in months.

Brian didn't want to lose this momentum. "Alright Mom, please tell me what you think is happening." He leaned forward in his chair again.

"Your Dad is here, Brian. That's all I know, and sometimes he takes me to where he is. I can't explain it so you'll understand it. Sometimes things just are not supposed to be explained. But if you will embrace this and stop fighting it, you will see him too. And then nothing, I mean absolutely nothing, will matter anymore other than this. All bad business decisions, all the people who cut you off in traffic, every judgment you have about others and yourself, none of it will matter. There is so much love where your Dad is and he shares it with me every now and then. I can't wait to see him all the time...to join him. But before I go I want you and Emma to believe and understand what I'm trying to tell you. You have to open your hearts to this."

"That's a big responsibility you're laying on me Mom," Brian lowered his eyes.

"It's really not, Brian. All you have to do is be open to the possibilities," Emma said. When she said that, Peter became very clear to her. He smiled at her and it sent chills up and down her entire body. "Oh, God!" she whispered, sitting straight back in her chair.

"What?" Brian asked as he looked at Emma. He could see a change in her; a peace about her he hadn't seen in a long time.

"It's really Dad, Brian, and I can *feel* him." Emma began to radiate with light. It was clear to Brian something was happening to her.

"Be open to the possibilities," Emma said at the same time as Sara. Sara was radiating the same light as Emma.

Brian looked at both of them and with desperation in his voice said, "I don't know how!"

Peter came to Brian's side and touched him on his shoulder. The intensity of the energy began to grow; slowly at first but with each moment there was more of a tingling sensation.

"I feel something on my shoulder…a tingling. Is that what you're talking about?" Brian asked Emma and Sara at the same time.

"Dad's touching you. I can see him. Yes, that's what we're talking about."

"I'm open to all possibilities. I'm open to all possibilities." Brian began to chant quietly to himself. Each time he spoke, the tingling grew a little. This fueled Brian and he began to chant with more intensity until his entire body began to tingle. It wasn't overwhelming, but it was inescapable.

"I feel him but I don't see him!"

"Baby steps, honey. Baby steps." Sara said.

Just inside the patio window, Jane and the other Shadow People were watching the exchange from outside. The light on the patio was so intense they wanted to run.

"This is too much for me. Look at those people! Just who do they think they are?" Jane asked.

"They are part of the Light of the World, little ones." It was Yesh. "You don't have to stay in the dark. You can come with us." He, Silas and Tara were standing behind them, quietly observing the exchange going on outside.

Jane turned at the sound of his voice and when she saw him she crumbled. All the anger left her and she knelt at his feet. "Oh my, please take me. Please forgive me. Please take me. Please forgive me," she said over and over.

"Yes Jane, we will take you. Stand up and come with us," Yesh said as he took her hand, helping her to rise to her feet. Immediately she vanished from the room.

The Shadow People who had been surrounding Hank took a few steps back. They weren't ready yet. "You may come too," Yesh said as he turned in their direction. But they backed away into the shadows where they had come from.

"To gather another day," Silas said with grin.

Yesh returned the smile and they left, content with the knowledge Jane was finally at peace and Peter was doing great work.

"You need to go now, I need my rest," Sara said to all on the patio. "I'm tired and want to take a nap."

She began to pull at her wheelchair. Brian stood, walked behind her and wheeled her in the house. He was full of energy and a peace he had never felt before. He didn't want this to go away.

"Thanks Em, you did great on your Very Important Mission," Peter said as he crouched next to Emily.

"I did do a good job, huh, and I'll do it again. Just let me know when!" She was doing pirouettes and moving towards the door. Buster stood beside her wagging his tail.

"Bye Dad," Emma said with tears in her eyes, as she took Emily's hand and walked towards the door.

"Bye sweetheart," Peter whispered in Emma's ear.

Chapter 24

Sara slept well for the first time in weeks. She had been exhausted from the visit with the family. Emma's, and especially Brian's, realization there was more to life than what they could see was amazing, but now Sara needed to rest.

Her vision was becoming clearer, less foggy and shapes appeared denser. She felt as though she was not in her body any longer because she saw herself floating along a dirt walkway. Trees on either side of her began to take shape, standing tall with their branches reaching up to the sky. She followed the tree line and saw red rocks up ahead. The more she looked ahead the clearer things became. She saw a beautiful mountain in front of her; bright red and brown colors surrounded it.

"That's Bell Rock! I'm in Sedona again!" she thought. *"Peter and I love this place. I remember the first time we hiked it. I was so afraid so I didn't go to the top. Peter went all the way and waved at me. He was so kind about my silly fears. I wish I had gone up there with him."*

Suddenly, feeling a gentle swoop, Sara found herself at the top of Bell Rock. She was a little off balance at first, adjusting to the sudden change in her surroundings but trying more to adjust to the trip itself. She found herself looking out over a vast expanse of red rocks. She noticed was there were no roads, no cars, no civilization.

"We are multidimensional beings, Sara." It was Matthew again, dressed as he had been the last time she had seen him. "Here, you can travel at the speed of thought."

"I've always loved this place and felt bad about how people had carved into the beauty. We would hike along the trail that was supposed to be peaceful but we could still hear the cars on the highway. Now I don't see any highway. In fact, I don't see any people at all."

Sara turned in a small circle, looking at all areas of the landscape. "Untouched. This is what untouched means, isn't it?"

"Untouched by humans, but not untouched by The Divine," Matthew said as he spread his arms out wide and up to the sky. "This is exactly how God created this place. He gave it to people and they did what they did with it. His gift is unconditional. What people do with it is up to them. Remember, He has no sadness or distaste for what has happened in the dimension you just came from."

"Ah, so where I 'just came from' as you say still has cars, houses, and all the carving into the landscape?" She turned to face him directly, looking up at his beautiful eyes. "By the way, I do like you dressing this way. It's very biblical and makes me feel like I'm safe."

"That's the point dear one. And yes, where you came from does still have cars and the rest. But, being multidimensional, you can come here merely by meditating, sitting quietly with your eyes closed, breathing in the Breath of The Divine. There are many ways to get to where we are. Your reason at this time is to escape your body. To leave the uncomfortable for the comfortable."

"So, if I think about my body I'll go back there?"

Sara was worried she would be in pain again. Here there was no pain; no discomfort at all. She was light and appeared to be 25 years old again. She had been in her best shape at that age.

"Matthew, please show me the way out of there."

"You are progressing in a sense, turning away from the body that no longer is of service to you, and moving in a direction that will bring you to the next phase of your existence. This is one of the phases. We observed your dream and assisted you to make it more lucid, more of an actual experience, if you will. You are on your way out of there, and on your way to somewhere. Everything is on its way somewhere. All creation is in constant movement, but the key is to get beyond doubt. To move forward we must not doubt the existence of The Divine.

"There are many who suffer needlessly with their struggle with being on the Earth plane. They feel they must make money, acquire possessions and beat down their neighbor or co-worker. They are in constant competition which is so unnecessary. Humans have created games that hurt one another and call it entertainment. This started long ago when the Romans had gladiators, and even before that. Humanity's aggression has only caused them to be further separated from The Divine. Again, peaceful conflict resolution gets Humans closer to The Divine. The Great Master, Jesus, said it best when He said, 'turn the other cheek.'"

"That has been something I've always tried to do and I know I've failed many times."

"And The Divine gives you continuous opportunities to master that emotion. That's all they are, opportunities to change the way you respond to a situation."

Sara was quiet for a while, enjoying the vision that was before her. She took a deep breath and sensed the aroma of the trees, earth and sky. It enveloped her entire being and she could feel herself becoming that which she sensed.

"We rely too much on our five senses don't we," she said as she felt the ground, felt the air, felt the sky.

"Yes. You can 'be' what you pay attention to. But it's time for you to go back now. They are preparing for you to cross permanently and you have one or two more things to do first." Matthew took her hand. As he did, she woke up in her bed.

Emma and Brian were in her room, with Pastor Paul. It was late in the evening and all the other residents had gone to sleep.

"Oh, Pastor Paul, how nice to see you," Sara smiled.

He was holding her hand and sitting on the edge of the bed. She woke up as she felt his touch. At first she thought she was holding Matthew's hand.

"Nice to see you too," he smiled. "You've been sleeping a while now. Emma and Brian called me to visit, and I'm glad I stopped by."

"I'm glad you did too. I was visiting with Matthew on the top of Bell Rock. It's so beautiful there. I think I might go back pretty soon," she squeezed his hand. He returned the squeeze with a knowing smile.

"I thought we could share some prayers and talk about what's happening to you. Would you like that?" he asked, always with compassion.

"I would. Thank you Pastor Paul. My favorite is The Lord's Prayer."

In a hushed voice, Pastor Paul bowed his head, took both of Sara's hands into his and quietly recited The Lord's Prayer. He whispered a few more, knowing at this point in Sara's transition, loud noises harmed her sense of peace.

Sara fell into another deep sleep, but not before reaching out for Emma and Brian. Pastor Paul stood, motioning them to the bed to take his place. Sara held each of their hands, kissing each one and smiled as she began to sleep again.

"Part of the dying experience is reduced appetite and weight loss as they begin to slow down," Dr. Sanchez had explained. "Your Mom's body doesn't need the food she once did. Those who are dying will sleep more. Her body now has an altered chemistry which gives her a mild sense of euphoria. She is neither hungry nor thirsty and she is not suffering in any way by not eating. It is an expected part of her journey."

"She may also experience hallucinations, sometimes seeing or speaking to people who aren't there. We know this has been going on for a long time now, so I'm not surprised at all by her observations. She may feel cold to the touch; her blood pressure will become lower and her pulse will be irregular, slowing or speeding up. Her skin color will change as her circulation becomes diminished. Her breathing will change. She may have a surge of energy where she may sit up on her own, or open her eyes and talk to you with complete clarity."

Doc. Sanchez was used to having this discussion with family. He thought Brian and Emma were taking it better than most family members.

Others would cry inconsolably, or ask questions pertaining to how to keep their loved one around. Brian and Emma did just the opposite. They nodded their heads in understanding while watching their mom. It was an acceptance he wished all the families had.

"Thank you for taking care of her," Emma said. She gave him a quick hug and sat back down in the chair by Sara. Brian stood and shook his hand, not really looking at him, not wanting to take his gaze away from her.

"I'll be back in to check on her from time to time," he said. "It won't be long now." He quietly closed the door behind him.

"If I could, you know I would let you go Mom. I think I'm ready now," Emma said quietly in Sara's ear. "So fade away. Go to the meadow with Dad."

Chapter 25

SARA MOVED THROUGH THE VEIL with ease now. She no longer struggled to see and as she released this need, her vision began to clear. The colors of the flowers and trees illuminated with brilliance. She took a step, and as she looked at her feet, she was young again. Her body had transformed itself. But it wasn't really a body. She was translucent; she held up her hand and saw through it to the sky. There was form, but it wasn't solid.

"Ah, so that's what you mean by being Light; by being 'of the Light.' I get it now." And as she took another step, everything behind her began to fade.

Sounds she never heard before began engulf her. She could hear the singing of a beautiful woman's voice, not singing words but an Angelic tune. The background sounds began to get louder. It was a chant, something similar to the one Emma had played for her while she was in the nursing home.

"*No, wait. This is the same music. Am I still in my room? Where is this beautiful place?*" she thought out loud.

As the music became louder, the Light became brighter. Birds of every species in pairs began to fly above, circling around her. Humming birds sat on her outstretched hand. She could hear a dog barking. As she looked around, she saw Tasha, her beloved black Labrador mix who had died years ago when she was a little girl.

"Tasha! Hey baby girl, how are you?" She knelt down to accept her.

Tasha came running up to her side and leaned her body on Sara. This was Tasha's way of hugging and it felt so good to see her again.

"Tasha, you've been gone for so long! Oh, I guess I must be dead, huh?" she looked around. "Well, if this is Heaven, then I'm glad to be in it!"

As she came to the realization of where she was, all of the animals who had ever kept her company her entire life began to emerge from the forest around her. Stardust, Dana, and other horses she had so long ago she couldn't remember their names, came trotting up from far off in a field. Numerous dogs and cats and the three bunnies she rescued decades ago began to follow each other to be by her side.

"*We've been waiting for you Mommy,*" Tasha thought. As she thought those words, Sara heard them. While it may have seemed strange before, Sara completely understood the ability to communicate with Tasha in those ways.

"I've missed you all so much!" Sara said sitting down on the grass next to the road in order to hold each of them. Tears began to stream down her face. "I love you all."

"*We love you too,*" they thought in unison. "*We have been with you always, we never left.*"

As Sara looked up from hugging Buster, the red dog who had been of service to her in the nursing home, she saw the shapes of people in the distance. They were engulfed in light and not easy to make out, but they began to move closer, and as they did they became clearer.

"*Go ahead Mommy,*" Tasha thought. "*They've been waiting for you too.*"

It was The Three, Yesh, Silas and Tera. They glided to her, and as they got closer they became more visible and seemed to take on the form of humans.

"Peter told me about you. You are The Three, aren't you?" Sara asked as she began to stand.

"Yes, dear one. We came to show you The Way," Yesh spoke with such peacefulness in his voice. It was more a thought than spoken words. Sara knew what he was about to tell her.

"Yes, Peter is up ahead of us. He assisted you in coming here, but it is our mission, if you will, to help you go to where he is now."

Yesh reached for her and took her hand. The energy coming from Yesh filled her light body and she began to glow as they did. A feeling of peace and love overwhelmed her and she began to cry.

Simultaneously, Yesh, Silas and Tera surrounded her and supported her. They held hands to elbows in a circle around her and projected a Light from their hearts into Sara. This was the same feeling, albeit much stronger, she had while travelling with Peter and Matthew. It was the same feeling she had on her shoulder when she felt alone and weary. Each time these Light Beings had touched her, she had felt comfort and peace. Now, more than ever, she felt it in her soul. Being without her physical body made it much easier to bring it to her heart. She no longer felt the denseness of her body, or the pain of the arthritis and confusion of the dementia. Because of this, she was able to absorb their Love and Peace and she began to glow.

"So this is what a Lightworker is," she said smiling.

"Yes," Tera thought. "This is how people on the Earth plane project our Light into one another."

"I want to do this," Sara replied. "How do I do this for others?"

"You are here now and as you absorb this, you will be able to project it to others on this plane and on the Earth plane. Just think it and it is done," Silas explained.

"I am filled with this Love and this Light. I've heard the term 'Love & Light' being wished to people instead of 'good day' but feeling it is different. Having the experience is different than learning about it. I am blessed to know and feel now."

"She's got it," Silas said and they broke the circle. As they did, the illumination of Sara stayed with her. All that surrounded her was now clear. Her very being was illumined and her expression transfixed into complete Peace and Love.

"She got it quicker than I did." It was Peter, standing behind Yesh.

"That's because she did the work on the Earth plane you had not." Yesh explained. "But it never matters how long it takes anyone, as you have learned. There is no time here, and no competition. Everyone evolves at their own pace. She was more open to the possibilities and needed to absorb less. We are all where we are supposed to be. Let's show her the rest of this place, yes?"

Peter held out his hand to Sara. She smiled sweetly, as she had the first day they met, and all of them walked towards the two suns shining on the horizon, with animals in tow.

About the Author

Rev. Susan Henley is the author of *Because of Sean, the True Story of a Mother's Courage*. She is an ordained Spiritual Peace Minister with The Beloved Community and Universal Life Church. As an ordained minister, she provides spiritual counseling in the areas of grief and loss with inspiration and encouragement when things seem at their worst. She helps her clients achieve direction towards advancement in harmony with career, relationships and home. Sue is an author, speaker, certified Spiritual Counselor and Reiki Master and regularly performs weddings, baptisms and funerals. She is a native of Arizona. Her dedication to her clients and their well being makes Sue a valuable asset to them and to the community. Sue is well known for her leadership of self-realization opportunities and for her participation in charity events.

CPSIA information can be obtained at www.ICGtesting.com
Printed in the USA
BVOW080643021112

304405BV00003B/4/P